Oral Medication and Insulin Therapies

A Practical Guide for Reaching Diabetes Target Goals

CHARLENE FREEMAN

D1041607

"I am fortunate to have had great diabetes education and your assistance, Charlene. Your book is easy to understand and the educational handouts with clinical target goals, action of insulin, sick day guidelines, and troubleshooting guide would be extremely beneficial for the patient with diabetes."

—Sue Staker
(Diabetes patient on an insulin pump)

"I have really gotten an education on diabetes. I especially liked the page for site rotations, the action of the insulin was superb and the insulin regimens chart was very helpful. This would be an excellent reference and I think you have done an outstanding work here."

—Marilyn Scharff, RN,
(Utilization Review/Case Manager at a medical center)

"It's a great writing. This is the kind of resource our IM/FM office would find very helpful, both for physicians and nurses. Just the troubleshooting guide alone would be as useful to our nurses as they answer questions by phone. It would make a great study for RN and LVN CEUs."

—Carolyn Hartman, RN
(Internal medicine/family medicine office nurse)

I read your book twice and of course learned both times. It is really concise and full of information! This is good information for nurses to understand why certain meds are given and handling patients and questions. Great Job!"

—Sally Hartman, RN,
(Short Surgical Stay Unit staff nurse)

"The prevention of diabetes is so important and most clinicians should integrate the information into the care of their patients. Family practice physicians and nurse practitioners need this type of information to assist in the care of their diabetes patients. Great resource!

—Phyllis Updike, BS, MSN, DNS
(Professor emeritus and nurse practitioner)

Oral Medication and Insulin Therapies

A Practical Guide
for
Reaching Diabetes Target Goals

CHARLENE FREEMAN

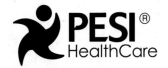

EAU CLAIRE, WISCONSIN
2008

PESI HealthCare, LLC
PO Box 900
200 Spring Street
Eau Claire, Wisconsin 54702

Printed in the United States of America

ISBN: 0-9722147-5-5

PESI HealthCare strives to obtain knowledgeable authors and faculty for its publications and seminars. The clinical recommendations contained herein are the result of extensive author research and review. Obviously, any recommendations for patient care must be held up against individual circumstances at hand. To the best of our knowledge any recommendations included by the author or faculty reflect currently accepted practice. However, these recommendations cannot be considered universal and complete. The author and publisher repudiate any responsibility for unfavorable effects that result from information, recommendations, undetected omissions or errors. Professionals using this publication should research other original sources of authority as well.

For information on this and other PESI HealthCare manuals and audio recordings, please call 800-843-7763 or visit our website at www.pesihealthcare.com

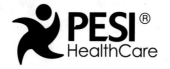

About the Author

Charlene Freeman, RN, CDE, CPT has had more than 30 years of diabetes patient management, diabetes program development, patient and educator training, development of clinical protocols, marketing materials, and has served as an independent consultant.

She developed and directed clinic-based diabetes education programs that have received American Diabetes Association (ADA) recognition and state accreditation, meeting the national standards for diabetes self-management education. Insulin pump therapy and multiple daily injection therapies are areas of particular interest and expertise to the speaker.

Ms. Freeman has presented over 1300 diabetes educational workshops to professionals, patients, and the public internationally, nationally, state-wide and locally. She was invited to co-chair workshops at the I.D.F. (International Diabetes Federation) at Kobe, Japan and present at Tokyo. Charlene is well respected as a diabetes educator.

She is past President, Health Care and Education of the national organization of the ADA and is past president of the Iowa Affiliate of the ADA.

Acknowledgements

The author wishes to give a heartfelt thanks to the following individuals who assisted with comments about this publication:

Carolyn Hartman, RN
Internal Medicine/Family Medicine office
Houston, Texas

Sally Hartman, RN
SSU (Short Surgical Stay Unit)
Ames, Iowa

Marilyn Scharff, RN
Utilization Review/Case Manager
Phelps Memorial Health Center
Holdredge, Nebraska

Sue Staker
Special Education instructor who was diagnosed with type 1 diabetes in 1991 and started insulin pump therapy 1996
Des Moines, Iowa

Phyllis Updike, BS, MSN, DNS
Community Health Nurse-Maternal and Child Health Professor Emeritus of University of Colorado Health Science Center
Dillon, Colorado

I dedicate this book to my husband, Judd Freeman, who has supported my career as a diabetes educator for more than thirty years. Our breakfast and dinner meals were frequently interrupted with calls from my diabetes patients needing assistance with their insulin dosage. He encouraged me during challenging times while on the national American Diabetes Association executive committee and continues to tolerate my numerous trips around the country.

Table of Contents

Table of Contents

Preface

Oral Medication and Insulin Therapies: A Practical Guide for Reaching Diabetes Target Goals is intended as a support for health care professionals who are assisting people with diabetes to reach target goals. The various oral medications and their mechanisms, as well as the types and regimens of the insulin are discussed. Reaching target goals has been shown to prevent the acute (hypoglycemia and hyperglycemia) and chronic (retinopathy, nephropathy, neuropathy, coronary heart disease and stroke) complications of diabetes.

Oral Medication and Insulin Therapies: A Practical Guide for Reaching Diabetes Target Goals provides guidelines to manage the medical needs of the patient with type 1 or 2 diabetes and is meant only as an estimated initiation guide that should be modified by patient experience and clinical judgment. Time course of action of any insulin can vary in different people, or at different times in the same person; thus, time periods indicated in this text should be considered general guidelines only. Self-Monitoring Blood Glucose (SMBG) before meals, 2 hours after meals, bedtime, and during the night is necessary to ascertain the action of oral medication and insulin for individual patients. The process of reaching target blood glucose (BG) usually requires at least four weeks with significant patient education (utilizing a nurse diabetes educator and dietitian diabetes educator) and coaching of self-management skills.

While every reasonable precaution has been taken in the preparation of this document, the author and publisher assume no responsibility for errors or omissions or for the uses made of the materials contained herein and the decisions based on such use. No warranties are made, expressed or implied, with regard to the contents of this document or to its applicability to specific individuals or circumstances. The author or the publisher shall not be liable for direct, indirect, special, incidental or consequential damages arising out of the use of or inability to use the contents of this manual. The author advises patients to always check with their physician/healthcare professional for advice on specific treatment of their diabetes.

Understanding Diabetes

1

Normal Metabolism

Diabetes still remains one of the leading causes of death in the United States because of the complications associated with this metabolic condition. These complications can be prevented by reaching target blood glucose (BG) goals.[1,2]

Pathophysiology should be understood by the health care professional, as well as the patient with diabetes, in order to comprehend all of the complexities that can alter BG results in diabetes. To begin to understand diabetes use **Figure 1: What is Normal Metabolism.**

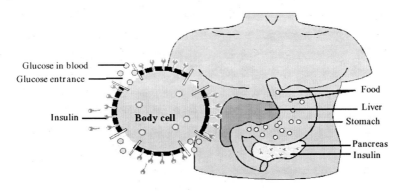

Figure 1: What is Normal Metabolism?

When **food** is eaten, it goes to the **stomach** and changes to **glucose (sugar)**. Everything eaten changes to glucose (even meat is 50% glucose).

Glucose stimulates the beta cells in the islets of Langerhans in the **pancreas** to give off **insulin**. Protein does not require insulin to be utilized.

Insulin is the **key** that opens the **doors (receptor sites)** on the cells to allow the glucose to enter the cell for **energy**.

Energy is needed every second of the day, but food is not eaten every second of the day. Extra glucose not used immediately for energy is stored in the **liver** as **glycogen** (or glucose). If more food is eaten than is burned for energy, that glucose is stored as fat.

Diabetes is a metabolic condition in which either the pancreas produces insufficient insulin or the body cells utilize glucose ineffectively. This results in abnormally elevated blood glucose (BG) levels that, if not controlled, lead to the debilitating complications of diabetes.

Hormones That Affect Blood Glucose

In addition to normal metabolism, **hormones** can alter the BG levels in patients with diabetes. Note **Figure 2: Hormones That Affect Blood Glucose (BG)**.

HORMONE	EFFECT ON BG
Insulin	▼
Amylin	▼
GLP-1	▼
Glucagon	▲
Epinephrine	▲
Glucocorticoids	▲
Growth Hormone	▲
Progesterone, HPL, Cortisol	▲

Figure 2: Hormones That Affect Blood Glucose (BG)

Insulin is normally secreted by the beta cells in the pancreas. Insulin helps to return plasma glucose concentrations to the fasting levels primarily by stimulating the uptake of glucose from the circulation into the muscle and fat cells for storage.

Amylin is also normally secreted by the beta cells in the pancreas. Amylin works as a partner hormone to insulin and glucagon, helping to regulate the post-meal increase in glucose concentrations.

Amylin manufactured as Symlin® (pramlintide):

- Slows gastric emptying

- Suppresses glucagon release

- Decreases appetite by causing a feeling of fullness

Trials indicate that amylin injections before meals may reduce the amount of injected insulin required by diabetes patients.

GLP-1 (glucagon-like peptide-1) is a gut derived hormone found to be decreased in Type 2 patients.

GLP-1 manufactured as Byetta® (exenatide):

- Slows gastric emptying, therefore decreasing post prandial blood glucose

- Suppresses glucagon release

- Decreases appetite

- Increases beta cell responsiveness to glucose

- Decreases hepatic glucose production

Byetta is given by injection twice daily. Trials indicate Type 2 patients have a weight loss.

Glucagon is normally secreted by the alpha cells in the pancreas to stimulate the liver to give off glycogen and raise BG levels when a meal is omitted or late.

Epinephrine comes from the adrenal medulla during stress. This also causes the liver to give off glycogen stores. Patients with diabetes demonstrate elevated BG levels during episodes of stress, illness, surgery, etc.

Glucocorticoids stimulate the liver to give off glycogen stores. Cortisol is normally secreted by the adrenal cortex as the long-term stressor causing elevated BG for the diabetes patient. BG can be elevated with interthecal injections, i.e. an injection into the knee of a patient with diabetes caused a BG >500. The patient was not aware that her BG might elevate and she thought something was wrong with her insulin pump. Another patient was given prednisone for asthma which precipitated overt diabetes.

Growth Hormone from the pituitary gland stimulates the liver to give off glycogen. This causes an elevated BG in diabetes patients. Children experience "roller coaster" BG levels during periods of growth and their BG levels can be challenging to control. Growth hormone is present in both children and adults and may produce the **Dawn Phenomenon (Figure 3).** During the night when all the glycogen stores in the muscle are used, growth hormone stimulates the liver to give off glycogen causing an elevated morning BG in patients with diabetes. Therefore, the HS (hour of sleep) BG is normal, the 3 AM BG is normal, and the morning BG is elevated.

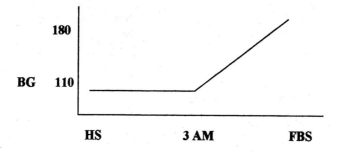

Figure 3: Dawn Phenomenon

Progesterone, HPL, and **Cortisol** are secreted by the placenta during pregnancy. Note **Figure 4: Insulin Requirements During Pregnancy.**[3] Human placenta lactogen (HPL), insulinase enzyme, and cortisol cause insulin resistance. Therefore, the amount of insulin required normally increases at 24–28 weeks gestation. This causes ges-

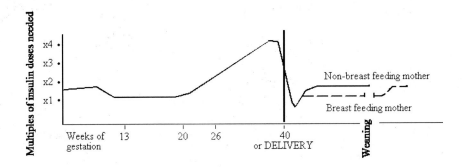

Figure 4: Insulin Requirements During Pregnancy

tational diabetes mellitus (GDM) if the beta cells in the pancreas cannot respond to the increased need for insulin. The woman with diabetes prior to pregnancy has a four-fold increase in insulin requirements during pregnancy. When the baby is born, the insulin requirements return to the non-pregnancy level.

Hormonal levels during menstrual period and menopause can also alter BG levels. Some patients with diabetes experience elevated BG levels five to ten days prior to menses and therefore, need more diabetes medication or insulin.

Classifications of Diabetes

A panel including members of the National Institutes of Health (NIH), Centers for Disease Control and Prevention (CDC), and American Diabetes Association (ADA) announced the Expert Committee Report in 1997. The report included classifications of diabetes to address the confusion surrounding Non-Insulin Dependent Diabetes Mellitus (NIDDM) patients who require insulin. The new classifications are:

- **Type 1 (Immune-mediated diabetes)** replaces Insulin-Dependent Diabetes Mellitus (IDDM) and Juvenile-onset Diabetes

- **Type 2 (Insulin-resistance)** replaces NIDDM and Mature-onset Diabetes
- **Impaired Glucose Homeostasis** or Pre-Diabetes includes:
  - **IFG (Impaired Fasting Glucose)** is a new category
  - **IGT (Impaired Glucose Tolerance)**
- **GDM (Gestational Diabetes Mellitus)** occurs during pregnancy.

Type I Diabetes Mellitus: Immune Mediated Diabetes

Type 1 diabetes is **immune mediated diabetes** and occurs when the beta cells in the pancreas are destroyed. Note **Figure 5: Type 1 Diabetes, Immune Mediated Diabetes.** The destruction of the pancreatic beta cells prevents the normal release of insulin and therefore, causes an abnormal increase in BG.

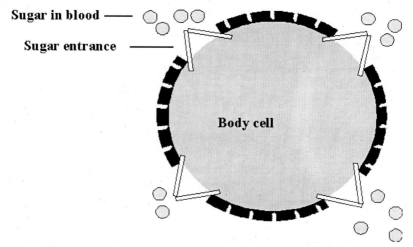

Figure 5: Type I Diabetes: Immune Mediated Diabetes

Many people have reported that type 1 diabetes developed after an episode of severe "flu." Although the onset may seem abrupt, beta cell destruction occurs over a variable interval of months to years and may be triggered by viral infections such as coxsackie B_4 and rubella. Beta cells are damaged by an autoimmune process in which the body produces antibodies against itself. Therefore, the new name "immune-mediated" is more correct and complete.

This classification was formerly called Insulin-Dependent Diabetes Mellitus (IDDM) as the patient "depends" on exogenous insulin injections to survive. The new classification is according to the etiology instead of the treatment of the condition.

This classification was also formerly known as Juvenile-onset Diabetes. Type 1 diabetes usually occurs before the age of 20. However, it can occur at a later age. Therefore, the term Juvenile-onset Diabetes is no longer used. The term **Latent Autoimmune Diabetes of Adulthood (LADA)** is now used to describe the condition in which adults acquire type 1 diabetes.

The classic symptoms of type 1 diabetes are:

- Polyuria (frequent urination)
- Polydipsia (increased thirst)
- Polyphagia (increased hunger)
- Unusual weight loss
- Extreme fatigue
- Irritability

When the beta cell in the pancreas secretes the insulin molecule, the C-peptide (connecting peptide) is cleaved off. The laboratory test to measure the amount of C-peptide in the serum ascertains if the amount of insulin is low (as in type 1 diabetes); or normal or elevated (as in type 2 diabetes). Note **Figure 6: Insulin Molecule with the C-Peptide.**

The diagnostic key to type 1 diabetes is that the patient is prone to **Diabetic Keto-Acidosis (DKA): Figure 7.** When there is not enough insulin to get the sugar into the cells for energy, fat is burned

7

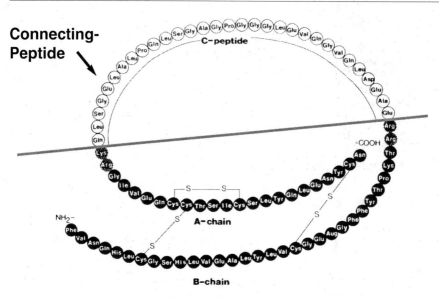

Connecting-Peptide

Figure 6: Insulin Molecule with the C-Peptide

for energy causing the body cells to become too acid, leading to DKA. This can lead to coma and death if not treated with insulin. DKA also occurs when the BG levels are too high in type 1 diabetes, especially when insulin is omitted.

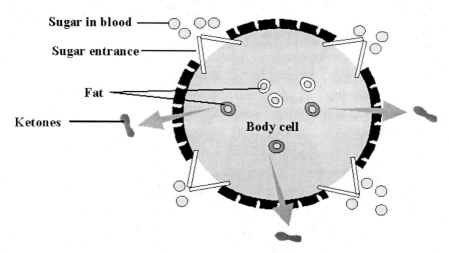

Figure 7: Diabetic Keto-Acidosis (DKA)

In summary, type 1 diabetes is:
• Auto-immune, islet cell antibodies present • Complete insulin deficiency (insulinopenic) • Absolute dependence upon exogenous insulin • Prone to DKA • Lean, recent weight loss • Abrupt onset, usually before age 40 • May occur in elderly

Type 2 Diabetes Mellitus: Insulin Resistance Diabetes

Type 2 diabetes is **insulin resistance diabetes** because the **doors (receptor sites)** on the cells close due to obesity, but the beta cells are not destroyed as in type 1. The pancreas continues to produce insulin, but a blockage occurs which prevents the body cells from utilizing BG. Ninety percent of type 2 diabetes patients are overweight or obese. Note **Figure 8: Type 2 Diabetes Mellitus: Insulin Resistance Diabetes.**

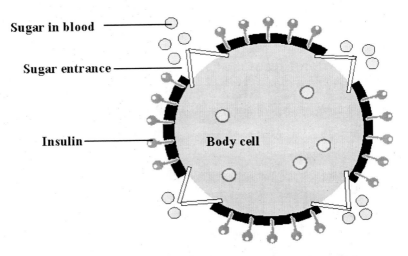

Sugar in blood

Sugar entrance

Insulin

Body cell

Figure 8: Type 2 Diabetes Mellitus: Insulin Resistance Diabetes

Type 2 was formerly known as Non-Insulin Dependent Diabetes Mellitus (NIDDM) and Mature-onset Diabetes. The name has been changed because many of these patients require insulin to reach target BG levels and type 2 can also occur at a younger age. Obesity and sedentary lifestyle are significant contributory influences to insulin resistance. In the US 65% of our population is overweight or obese. Type 2 diabetes is presently in epidemic proportions because increasing numbers of children are overweight, obese and inactive. Type 2 diabetes increased in youth 125% during 2002.

The symptoms of type 2 diabetes are:

- Any symptoms of type 1 diabetes
- Frequent infections
- Blurred vision
- Cuts/bruises slow to heal
- Tingling or numbness in hands/feet
- Recurring skin, gum, or vaginal/bladder infection
- No symptoms

Figure 9: Pathophysiology of Type 2 Diabetes shows the various areas that cause the hyperglycemia (elevated BG):

1. During the night the liver gives off an excess of glycogen or **increased hepatic glucose output** leading to elevated Fasting Blood Sugar (FPG) in the morning.

2. Insulin resistance due to receptor and post-receptor cell defects thought to be due to obesity causes **decreased peripheral glucose uptake** at the muscle leading to elevated BG before meals (AC).

3. Insulin deficiency due to **decreased insulin secretion** from the beta cell leading to elevated BG two hours postprandial or after eating (2 H PC).

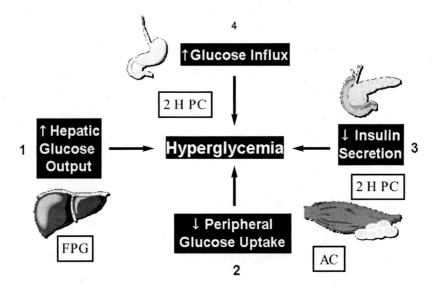

Figure 9: Pathophysiology of Type 2 Diabetes

4. Too much food causes **increased glucose influx**. This leads to elevated BG 2 H PC.

Note **Figure 10: Natural History of Type 2 Diabetes.**[4] The natural history of type 2 diabetes is illustrated more graphically in this figure. In the period preceding the onset of frank diabetes (characterized by impaired glucose tolerance) macrovascular risk (cardiovascular disease (CVD), coronary artery disease (CAD), peripheral vascular disease (PVD) and stroke (CVA)) is already very pronounced **(note large lower arrow)**. Microvascular risk (retinopathy, nephropathy, and neuropathy) begins after the onset of hyperglycemia.

The two lower graph lines illustrate fasting and postprandial (after eating) glycemia; the earliest abnormality in patients with type 2 diabetes is primarily observed in the postprandial state **(note large upper arrow)**. This abnormality remains more significant than the fasting plasma glucose abnormality for the duration of the disease.

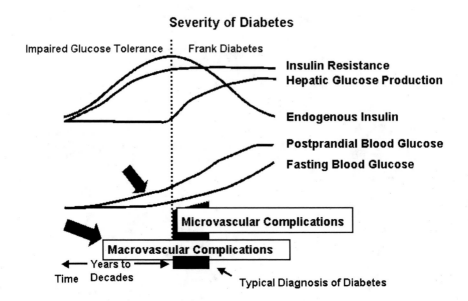

Figure 10: Natural History of Type 2 Diabetes

The fasting plasma glucose concentration begins to rise after the postprandial rise in glucose and is coincident with the increase in hepatic glucose production, which, in turn, is coincident with the decline of endogenous insulin secretion. Insulin resistance, which is fully expressed in the stage of impaired glucose tolerance, tends not to change very much over the course of disease. The insulin resistance causes **hyperinsulinemia** (increased endogenous insulin levels and C-peptide in the blood).

From this pathophysiologic scheme of progressive beta-cell failure, it is clear that over time all type 2 patients will require either increased endogenous insulin production or exogenous insulin therapy.

Note **Figure 11: Loss of 1st-Phase Insulin Secretion in Type 2 Diabetes.**[5] The left figure shows phases of insulin release based on the IV Glucose Tolerance Test (GTT) in normal subjects.

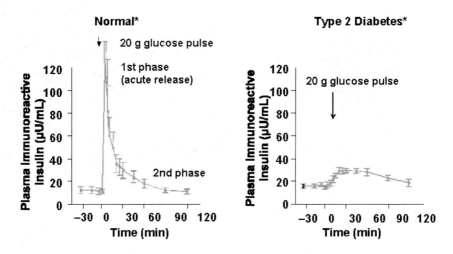

Figure 11: Loss of 1st-Phase Insulin Secretion in Type 2 Diabetes

- The 1st-phase (acute release) depends on immediate-releasable insulin stores, reflected as a sharp increase in insulin response in the first ten minutes.
- The 2nd-phase partially depends on insulin stores and protein synthesis within the beta cell, shown as persistent increase in insulin concentration from ten to one hundred twenty minutes.

The right figure shows the loss of 1st- and 2nd-release insulin secretion based on IV GTT in patients with type 2 diabetes. The loss of release of insulin secretion represents one of the earliest detectable manifestations; no clinically evident disease exists without this defect, despite presence of insulin resistance. Therefore, the BG 2 H PC is elevated.

Normal vs. type 2 diabetes		
Insulin Levels	**Normal**	**Type 2 Diabetes**
After glucose	↑ >7-fold	↓ 2-fold
Peak	within few min	~20 min
Decline	within min after peaking	60 min
Reach baseline levels	within 45 min	>120 min

13

"Syndrome X" or Metabolic Syndrome or Cardiometabolic Syndrome may be associated with insulin resistance, compensatory hyperinsulinemia, obesity (abdominal or visceral), dyslipidemia (elevated triglycerides, decreased HDL, elevated LDL) and hypertension. Syndrome X may have an increased rate of coronary heart disease (CHD). According to Dr. DeFronzo of San Antonio, the treatment for Syndrome X is 3 fold: exercise, exercise, and exercise! Weight loss, exercise and oral medication can decrease the resistance of the cells to insulin action.

In summary type 2 diabetes is:

- Not absolutely dependent upon exogenous insulin
- Progressive condition, gradual onset
- May be relatively free of classical symptoms
- Not prone to DKA
- Strong family history of diabetes mellitus
- Usually obese or history of obesity, sedentary lifestyle
- Usually diagnosed after age 40, but epidemic in youth
- Higher incidence in African-American, Hispanic-American, Native-American, Asian-American, Pacific Islander

---

Impaired Glucose Homeostasis or Pre-Diabetes

Impaired Glucose Homeostasis includes **Impaired Fasting Glucose (IFG)** and **Impaired Glucose Tolerance (IGT)**. These terms refer to a metabolic stage intermediate between normal glucose homeostasis and diabetes, now referred to as **"Pre-diabetes."** Impaired Glucose Tolerance (IGT) was formerly called "borderline diabetes." These patients are at potential risk for developing the chronic complications of diabetes and Coronary Heart Disease (CHD).[6]

Gestational Diabetes Mellitus

Gestational diabetes mellitus (GDM) is defined as any degree of glucose intolerance with onset or first recognition during pregnancy, (Note **Figure 4: Insulin Requirements During Pregnancy**). The definition applies regardless of whether insulin or only diet modification is used for treatment or whether the condition persists after pregnancy. Forty to sixty percent of gestational diabetes patients will develop overt type 2 diabetes in 7 to 10 years post partum. If they are lean and fit, the risk factor is 25%. The chance of developing type 1 within one year is 3–7%.

Risk Factors and Diagnosis of Diabetes Mellitus

2

Risk Factors for Diabetes Mellitus

All patients should be screened for type 2 diabetes mellitus after age 45. The BG 2 H PC (2 hour post prandial BG) is elevated prior to the Fasting Plasma Glucose (FPG) or Fasting Blood Sugar (FBS) exhibiting abnormal BG levels in diabetes patients. Testing should be done at a younger age, or carried out more frequently, in individuals who have the following risk factors for diabetes.

Risk Factors for diabetes are:

- have first-degree relative with diabetes
- exhibit obesity: $\geq$ 120% desirable body weight or $\geq$ 25 Body Mass Index (BMI)

  Normal BMI: 18.5–24.9
  Overweight: 25–29.9
  Obese: >30

Note **Figure 12: Body Mass Index Chart (BMI)**

- had IGT or IFG on previous testing
- is a member of high-risk ethnic population: African-American, Hispanic-American, Native-American, Asian-American, Pacific Islander
- are habitually physically inactive
- are hypertensive: > 140/90
- have an HDL cholesterol ≤ 35 or triglyceride ≥ 250
- have polycystic ovary syndrome
- have delivered baby > 9 lb. or have been diagnosed with GDM
- have a history of vascular disease[6]

Screening those at risk for diabetes is important, not only for identifying those who are unaware that they have overt diabetes, but also because the Diabetes Prevention Program (DPP) for type 2 demonstrated that this category of diabetes can be prevented.[6] The study compared counseling patients to make lifestyle changes (medical nutrition therapy/exercise and behavior modification) to medication. In this study the risk of developing type 2 diabetes was **decreased by 58%** with the following:

- The patients exercised thirty minutes five times each week.
- Dietary fat was reduced to <25% of the total calories per day.
- The patients had a modest weight loss of 5%–7% of their body weight.

The study also demonstrated that counseling patients to make the above lifestyle changes was more effective than Metformin medication in preventing type 2 diabetes.

This highlights the importance of utilizing a diabetes nurse educator and dietitian diabetes educator to coach self-management skills, not only for patients with overt diabetes, but also to prevent the acquisition of diabetes in other patients. This can be especially effective in those patients exhibiting impaired glucose homeostasis which includes Impaired Fasting Glucose (IFG) and Impaired Glucose Tolerance (IGT).

Body Mass Index Table

BMI	Normal						Overweight					Obese										Extreme Obesity															
	19	20	21	22	23	24	25	26	27	28	29	30	31	32	33	34	35	36	37	38	39	40	41	42	43	44	45	46	47	48	49	50	51	52	53	54
Height (inches)																Body Weight (pounds)																				
58	91	96	100	105	110	115	119	124	129	134	138	143	148	153	158	162	167	172	177	181	186	191	196	201	205	210	215	220	224	229	234	239	244	248	253	258
59	94	99	104	109	114	119	124	128	133	138	143	148	153	158	163	168	173	178	183	188	193	198	203	208	212	217	222	227	232	237	242	247	252	257	262	267
60	97	102	107	112	118	123	128	133	138	143	148	153	158	163	168	174	179	184	189	194	199	204	209	215	220	225	230	235	240	245	250	255	261	266	271	276
61	100	106	111	116	122	127	132	137	143	148	153	158	164	169	174	180	185	190	195	201	206	211	217	222	227	232	238	243	248	254	259	264	269	275	280	285
62	104	109	115	120	126	131	136	142	147	153	158	164	169	175	180	186	191	196	202	207	213	218	224	229	235	240	246	251	256	262	267	273	278	284	289	295
63	107	113	118	124	130	135	141	146	152	158	163	169	175	180	186	191	197	203	208	214	220	225	231	237	242	248	254	259	265	270	278	282	287	293	299	304
64	110	116	122	128	134	140	145	151	157	163	169	174	180	186	192	197	204	209	215	221	227	232	238	244	250	256	262	267	273	279	285	291	296	302	308	314
65	114	120	126	132	138	144	150	156	162	168	174	180	186	192	198	204	210	216	222	228	234	240	246	252	258	264	270	276	282	288	294	300	306	312	318	324
66	118	124	130	136	142	148	155	161	167	173	179	186	192	198	204	210	216	223	229	235	241	247	253	260	266	272	278	284	291	297	303	309	315	322	328	334
67	121	127	134	140	146	153	159	166	172	178	185	191	198	204	211	217	223	230	236	242	249	255	261	268	274	280	287	293	299	306	312	319	325	331	338	344
68	125	131	138	144	151	158	164	171	177	184	190	197	203	210	216	223	230	236	243	249	256	262	269	276	282	289	295	302	308	315	322	328	335	341	348	354
69	128	135	142	149	155	162	169	176	182	189	196	203	209	216	223	230	236	243	250	257	263	270	277	284	291	297	304	311	318	324	331	338	345	351	358	365
70	132	139	146	153	160	167	174	181	188	195	202	209	216	222	229	236	243	250	257	264	271	278	285	292	299	306	313	320	327	334	341	348	355	362	369	376
71	136	143	150	157	165	172	179	186	193	200	208	215	222	229	236	243	250	257	265	272	279	286	293	301	308	315	322	329	338	343	351	358	365	372	379	386
72	140	147	154	162	169	177	184	191	199	206	213	221	228	235	242	250	258	265	272	279	287	294	302	309	316	324	331	338	346	353	361	368	375	383	390	397
73	144	151	159	166	174	182	189	197	204	212	219	227	235	242	250	257	265	272	280	288	295	302	310	318	325	333	340	348	355	363	371	378	386	393	401	408
74	148	155	163	171	179	186	194	202	210	218	225	233	241	249	256	264	272	280	287	295	303	311	319	326	334	342	350	358	365	373	381	389	396	404	412	420
75	152	160	168	176	184	192	200	208	216	224	232	240	248	256	264	272	279	287	295	303	311	319	327	335	343	351	359	367	375	383	391	399	407	415	423	431
76	156	164	172	180	189	197	205	213	221	230	238	246	254	263	271	279	287	295	304	312	320	328	336	344	353	361	369	377	385	394	402	410	418	426	435	443

Source: Adapted from *Clinical Guidelines on the Identification, Evaluation, and Treatment of Overweight and Obesity in Adults: The Evidence Report.*

Figure 12: Body Mass Index Chart

Risk factors for type 2 diabetes in children age 10 or puberty:[6]

- Overweight (BMI >85%)
- Plus any 2 of the following:
  - Family history of type 2 diabetes
  - Non-Caucasian
  - Maternal history of diabetes or gestational diabetes
  - Signs or conditions of insulin resistance:
    -Acanthosis nigricans
    -Hypertension
    -Dyslipidemia
    -PCOS (Polycystic Ovary Syndrome)

Diagnosis of Diabetes Mellitus

The guidelines for the diagnosis of Diabetes Mellitus: (non-pregnant adult) are one of the following:[6]

- FPG (fasting > 8 hours) $\geq$ 126 mg/dL
- Random BG $\geq$ 200 mg/dL w/symptoms
- OGTT (Oral Glucose
  Tolerance Test: 75-g glucose) $\geq$ 200 mg/dL in 2 hr sample

Results must be confirmed on a subsequent day.

The guidelines for the diagnosis of **Impaired Glucose Homeostasis or Pre-Diabetes** (formerly called Borderline Diabetes) including IFG and IGT are:

Impaired Fasting Glucose (IFG):
FPG $\geq$ 100 mg/dl but < 126 mg/dL

Impaired Glucose Tolerance (IGT):
FPG $\geq$ 100 mg/dl but < 126 mg/dL
2 H PC $\geq$ 140 mg/dl but < 200 mg/dL[6]

Gestational Diabetes (GDM) screening is done between 24 and 28 weeks gestation because of the insulin resistance that occurs during pregnancy. (Note **Figure 4: Insulin requirements during pregnancy**).

Those at risk for GDM:[6]
- are older than age of 25
- exhibit obesity: $\geq$ 120% desirable body weight or $\geq$ 27 BMI

- have family history of diabetes
- have personal history of GDM
- exhibit glycosuria (glucose in the urine)
- are member of high-risk ethnic population: African-American, Hispanic-American, Native-American, Asian-American, Pacific Islander
- have previous unsuccessful pregnancy

Criteria for GDM:[6]

First Step: **Screen** with 50 g glucose challenge test (GCT)

- Usually given between 24–28 weeks.
- If 1-hr value is $\geq$ 200 mg/dL, diagnosis of GDM is made.
- If 1-hr value is $\geq$ 140 mg/dL, but $\leq$ 200 an oral glucose tolerance test (OGTT) should be performed as soon as possible, however the BG result of > 130–140 mg/dL will identify 80–90% of women with GDM.

Second Step: **Diagnose** with 100 g OGTT

- 2 abnormal values must be met or exceeded for diagnosis.
- Plasma glucose values (mg/dL):

  FPG $\geq$ 95
  1 hr pp $\geq$ 180
  2 hr pp $\geq$ 155
  3 hr pp $\geq$ 140

Clinical Target Goals for Diabetes

3

Clinical Target Goals for Diabetes: Blood Glucose and A_{1c}

Research has shown that reaching **target BG** and glycosylated hemoglobin A_{1c} (**A_{1c}**) is needed to prevent the long term complications of type 1 and type 2 diabetes or prevent the progression of the long term complications of type 1 diabetes:[1, 2, 6]

- retinopathy leading to blindness
- nephropathy leading to End Stage Renal Disease (ESRD) or kidney failure
- neuropathy and peripheral vascular disease (PVD) leading to amputation
- cardiovascular disease (CVD), coronary artery disease (CAD), and stroke (CVA)

Clinical target BG and A_{1c} goals should be determined for each individual diabetes patient.[6, 7, 8, 9] Note **Figure 13: Clinical Target Goals for Diabetes: BG and A_{1c}.** Target goals are different for the various life stages and for patients in high risk occupations. The goals are listed in both plasma and whole blood values since newer SMBG meters convert to plasma values.

Note the lower target BG goals during pre-conception and pregnancy. Close monitoring prior to and throughout pregnancy is crucial to prevent the complications to the fetus and the mother who has diabetes.

The target BG goals are different for children than for adults. The brain has its largest growth during the first five years of age. The target goals are set higher for children up to age thirteen to prevent unconscious or severe hypoglycemia and the resulting brain damage that might occur.[7]

The target BG goals are also set higher for the elderly because unconscious hypoglycemia can precipitate a stroke.

Patients working in some high risk occupations may need higher target goals to prevent severe hypoglycemia. Two examples of such occupations are heavy equipment operators and steel workers.

Some diabetes patients experience no symptoms for hypoglycemia (hypoglycemia unawareness). The target BG goals for these patients are set higher to prevent severe hypoglycemia from hypoglycemia unawareness.[1,6] Awareness of hypoglycemia can return by preventing any hypoglycemia for 48 hours.

Figure 13: Clinical Target Goals for Diabetes: BG and A_{1c} may be used as an educational hand-out for patients to understand their target BG goals. Making the diabetes patient aware of target BG can help improve adherence to diabetes management and assist the patient to learn self-management skills.

CLINICAL TARGET GOALS FOR DIABETES: BLOOD GLUCOSE & A$_{1c}$

Target BG (Individualize)	Non-diabetes	Goal	Take Action
Non-Pregnancy			
PLASMA VALUES (mg/dl)			
Average Premeal	<110	70–130	<70, >150
Average Bedtime	<120	110–150	<110, >180
2 hours after start of meal	<140	<160	>180
A$_{1c}$ (%)	<6	<7	>7
(Without risk of severe hypoglycemia)			
Pregnancy			
Premeal		60–105	≥105
1 hour after start of meal		≤ 155	≥155
2 hours after start of meal		≤ 130	≥130
Bedtime and 0200–0600		60–100	<60, >160
A$_{1c}$ (%)	<6	<6	>6
5th International GDM Conference:			
Premeal		≤ 90–99	
1 hour post-meal		≤ 140	
2 hours post-meal		≤ 120–127	
Pre-conception			
Premeal		70–100	
2 hours after start of meal		≤ 140	
A$_{1c}$ (%)		<1 above normal	
Hospital Management			
Premeal		<110	
2 hours after start of meal		<140	
Critically ill surgical patient		80–110	
Exceptions			
Children, elderly, chronic disease, CVD, high-risk occupation, hypoglycemic unawareness, history of severe hypoglycemia		100–200	<100, >200

For Youth	0–6 yrs	6–12 yrs	13–19 yrs
Premeal	100–180	90–180	90–130
2–3 hours after start of meal	<200	<200	<180
Bedtime	100–200	100–180	90–150
2–4 AM	>100	>100	>90
A$_{1c}$ (%)	>7.5 – <8.5	<8.0	<7.5

Figure 13: Clinical Target Goals for Diabetes: BG and A$_{1c}$

25

Management of Type 2 With Oral Medications

4

Management of Type 2 Diabetes Mellitus

Diabetes management includes: meal planning, Self-Monitoring Blood Glucose (SMBG), activity, education of diabetes and self-management skills, and medication therapy includes oral medications and insulin therapy. Note **Figure 14: Diabetes Management.** Only the medical management with oral medications and insulin therapy will be discussed in this publication.

Oral Medications for Type 2 Diabetes

Figure 15: Oral Medications for Type 2 Diabetes lists the various classifications of drugs, dosage, action, and therapeutic considerations.[9] Management should begin with the starting dosage and increase to maximum dosage. Note the therapeutic considerations and laboratory testing that needs to be done.

DIABETES MANAGEMENT

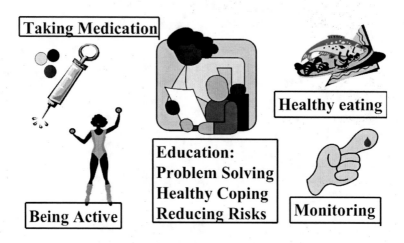

Figure 14: Diabetes Management

Matching Pharmacology to Pathophysiology

Determine which pathophysiologic mechanism is occurring by checking BG results and match the appropriate pharmacologic agent(s). **Figure 16: Matching Pharmacology to Pathophysiology** shows the medication of choice for each pathological mechanism that occurs in type 2 diabetes.

1. **Increased hepatic glucose output** (elevated FBS) = Biguanides, TZD, Insulin (bedtime NPH, Lantus or Levemir), Byetta® injections.

2. **Decreased peripheral glucose uptake** at the muscle (elevated BG AC) = TZD, Biguanides, Insulin (primarily basal insulin discussed later)

3. **Decreased insulin secretion** (elevated BG 2 H PC) = Sulfonylureas, Meglitinides, Insulin (primarily rapid-acting insulin discussed later), Byetta® injections

4. **Increased glucose influx** (elevated BG 2 H PC = Alpha-Glucosidase inhibitors

28

Staged Algorithm for Type 2 Diabetes Medical Management

Figure 17: Staged Algorithm for Type 2 Diabetes summarizes the algorithm for reaching glycemic control for the type 2 diabetes patient.[10] When the BG is above normal and the diagnosis of diabetes is made, then the A_{1c} will also assist to determine which therapy should be used. Note the % lowering of A_{1c} on the algorithm chart.

1. The consensus is that lifestyle intervention should be initiated as the first step in treating new-onset Type 2 diabetes.[10] Medical Nutrition Therapy should be implemented by a dietitian (preferably a CDE-Certified Diabetes Educator) utilizing Carbohydrate (CHO) Counting with weight management and an activity plan. This would also include diabetes education with SMBG. "The authors recognize that for most individuals with Type 2 diabetes, lifestyle interventions fail to achieve or maintain metabolic goals, either because of failure to lose weight, weight regain, progressive disease or a combination of factors."[10] Therefore, metformin therapy should be initiated concurrent with lifestyle intervention at diagnosis. (*See* **Figure 15: Oral Medications for Type 2**)

2. **Step 2** is adding <u>one</u> of the following medications to metformin if the A_{1c} goal is not achieved. Begin with the starting dose and increase to maximum dose:

   • Add basal insulin (bedtime NPH, or bedtime or morning Lantus® or Levemir®)-initiate with 10 units or 0.2 units/kg

   • Add TZD

   • Add SU (sulfonylurea or secretagogue)

If glycemic target goals are not achieved proceed to **Step 3,** and make further adjustments.

ORAL MEDICATIONS FOR TYPE 2

Trade name (how supplied)	Generic name	Starting dose (mg)	Max /day	Action	Therapeutic considerations
2nd Generation Sulfonylureas					
Amaryl (1, 2, 4)	Glimepiride	1-2 (1X/day)	8	Works to ▲output of insulin by beta cells in pancreas	Amaryl: Take with first main meal, less potential for low blood sugar, may reduce blood sugar faster. Can combine with all other drug classes. **Main potential side effect: hypoglycemia** with delayed or skipped meals, or alcohol. Use with caution in elderly patients. Metabolize by liver, excreted in urine and bile. No sulfa allergy reaction in patients with sulfa allergies. *Best taken 30 minutes prior to meal.
Glucotrol* (5, 10)	Glipizide	2.5, 10 (1-2X/day)	40		
Glucotrol XL (2.5, 5, 10)	Glipizide	5, 10	20		
Glynase Prestab* (1.5, 3, 6)	Glyburide	1.5 (0.75), 3 (w/ main meal)	12 qd (or 6 mg-bid)		
DiaBeta* Micronase* (1.25, 2.5, 5)	Glyburide	1.25-5	20 (or bid if >10)		
Insulin Secretagogues-Glinides					
Prandin (0.5, 1, 2)	Repaglinide	0.5, 1, 2 (ac each meal)	16 (4-qid)	Post-meal BG ▼ by causing ▲insulin-β-cell	Best taken 15-30 minutes before EACH meal. Can cause less hypoglycemia than Sulfonylurea as the action of this drug class is glucose level dependent. Can combine with all other drug classes. Prandin more effective at ↓ A$_{1c}$.
Starlix (60, 120)	Nateglinide	60, 120 (ac each meal)	360 (120-tid)		
Biguanide					
Glucophage (500, 850, 1000)	Metformin	500-850 tid or 1000 bid Peds: (10-16 yrs) 500 bid; Max: 2000	2550 (tid if >2g/day)	▼ liver output of sugar and ▲ peripheral insulin sensitivity	**Kidney surveillance testing required** (serum creatinine levels ≥1.5 (males), ≥1.4 mg/dL (females). **Contraindicated** if patient has CHF, ETOH abuse, metabolic acidosis, liver, or kidney disease, or ≥80 yrs old. Can combine with all other drug classes. May contribute to wt. loss. **Main potential side effects: GI distress/diarrhea; lactic acidosis.** Discontinue after OR, dye studies for 48 hrs or until kidney function normal. To minimize side effects start with low dose and titrate dose slowly. Take with food. When used alone does not cause hypoglycemia.
Glucophage XR (500, 750)	Metformin	500-2000 w/ evening meal	2000		
Fortamet XR (500,1000)			2500		
Glumetza XR (500-1000)			2000		
Riomet 500/5mL	(liquid Metformin)	500/5mL bid Peds: 2000	Adults: 2500		

Thiazolidinedione (TZD)

Brand (dose)	Generic			Mechanism	Notes
Avandia (2, 4, 8)	Rosigloitazone	2, 4, 8 Mono-therapy- 2-bid or 4 qd	4-bid or 8 qd Mono-therapy-8 Combination-4	▲ peripheral insulin sensitivity and ▼ liver output of sugar	**Liver function required initially, then prn. Avoid if ALT >2.5X ULN. Can cause fluid retention, exacerbate or lead to HF. If Class 1 or 2 HF-start low, ↑ slowly.** May take 4 months for full effect to be seen. Does not increase insulin production. When used alone or in combination with Metformin will not cause hypoglycemia. Approved for use with insulin and all other oral medications. Can improve fertility. Improves blood lipid levels.
Actos (15, 30, 45)	Pioglitazone	15, 30	Mono-therapy-45 Combination-30		

Combinations

Brand	Generic	Dose	Max
Actoplus met	Pioglitazone/Metformin	15/500, 15/850 daily or bid	45/2550
Avandamet	Rosiglitazone/Metformin	1/500, 2/500, 4/500, 2/1000, 4/1000	8/2000
Avandaryl	Rosiglitazone/ Glimepiride	4/1, 4/2, 8/4	8/4
Duetact	Pioglitazone/glimepiride	30/2,30/4	30/4
Glucovance	Glyburide/Metformin	1.25/250, 2.5/500, 5/500	20/2000
Metaglip	Metformin/Glipizide	250/2.5, 500/2.5, 500/5	1000/10 or 2000/20 (given bid)
Janumet	Januvia/Metformin	50/500, 50/1000	

Incretin Mimetics

Brand (dose)	Generic			Mechanism	Notes
Byetta (5mcg,10mcg)	Exenatide	5mcg SQ	10mcg bid	Mimics GLP1	Take w/ 20 min ac 2 major meals, then ↑ to 60 min ac. ↑ satiety, ↓ weight. Side effect: nausea.
Januvia (25,50,100)	Sitagliptin	25 mg	100	DPP4 inhibitor, ▲ GLP1	Januvia: do not take if renal insufficiency. Does not ↓ weight.
Symlin (60, 120 pens)	Pramlintide	60 mcg SQ ac	120 mcg ac	Mimics Amylin	Symlin: Use w/ insulin; ↓ meal insulin 50%, ↑ satiety, ↓ weight. Side effect: nausea.

This document is a guideline for the medical management of the patient with Type 2 diabetes and is meant only as an estimated initiation guide that should be modified by patient experience and clinical judgment. The process usually requires at least four weeks with significant patient education (utilizing a diabetes nurse educator and dietitian diabetes educator) and coaching of self-management skills.

Figure 15: Oral Medications for Type 2 (Continued)

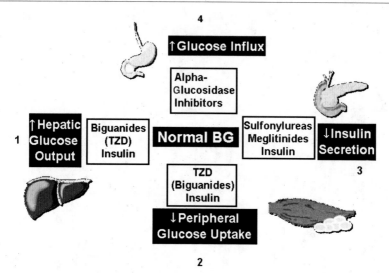

Figure 16: Matching Pharmacology to Pathophysiology

3. Addition of a third oral agent could be considered; however, this approach is relatively more costly and potentially not as effective in lowering glycemia compared with adding or intensifying insulin.

   • Metformin, SU, and /or TZD

   • Continue SU and/or Metformin and/or TZD and add bed-time insulin with NPH, Lantus®, or Levemir®

   • Insulin therapy: discontinue SU and initiate split-mixed dose or MDI (Multiple Daily Injections), continue TZD and/or Metformin

   • If Metformin is contraindicated, add basal insulin (Lantus® or Levemir®), taper off SU, and introduce bolus (rapid-acting insulin as needed).

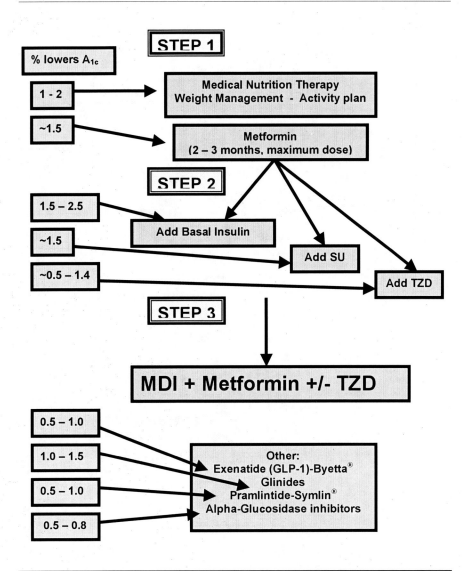

This document is a guideline for the medical management of the patient with Type 2 diabetes and is meant only as an estimated initiation guide that should be modified by patient experience and clinical judgment. The process usually requires at least four weeks with significant patient education (utilizing a diabetes nurse educator and a dietitian diabetes educator) and coaching of self-management skills.

Figure 17: Staged Algorithm for Type 2 Diabetes

The algorithm for the forced-titration schedule of **basal insulin** (either **Glargine-Lantus or NPH) added to oral therapy** is: [11]
Start with 10 U/day HS basal insulin dose and adjust weekly:

If SMBG-FPG (mg/dL)*	Increase in insulin dose (U/day)
≥180	8
≥140 but <180	6
≥120 but <140	4
≥100 but <120	2

Treat to target FPG ≤ 100 mg/dL

- *Patients should do SMBG fasting (FPG) for 2 consecutive days and experience no episodes of symptomatic nocturnal hypoglycemia (documented by FPG levels ≤72 mg/dL) or severe hypoglycemia (requiring the assistance of another person and confirmed by FPG <56 mg/dL) with insulin levels titrated until the target FPG of 100 mg/dL is reached.

- Patients with symptomatic hypoglycemia (SMBG FPG levels ≤72 mg/dL) should receive cessation of titration for 1 week, while those patients with severe hypoglycemia (SMBG FPG levels <56 mg/dL) should decrease 2–4 U/day of insulin to adjust the FPG levels.

- Reassess A_{1c} every 3 months until <7%, then every 6 months.

4. **Other medications:**
  - Exenatide (GLP-1, Byetta®)
    - 5 mcg/dose is injected bid within 60-minute period before morning and evening meals (or before two main meals of the day, approximately 6 hours or more apart).
    - Increase to 10 mcg bid after 2 months of therapy, if necessary.

- Glinides (Prandin® and Starlix®) "Prandin® is more effective at lowering A_{1c} than Starlix®."[10]
- Pramlintide (Amylin, Smylin®)(injection added to insulin therapy)
  - Reduce mealtime insulin by 50% when Symlin® is initiated.
  - Begin with 10 units (60μ) prior to meals (at least 250 calories or 30 grams of CHO).
  - Increase dosage to 20 units (120μ) when there has been no nausea for 3 or more days.
- Alpha-Glucosidase inhibitors

Insulin Therapy: Types of Insulin

5

Normal Insulin Action

To maintain euglycemia (non-diabetes BG) the pancreas normally secretes a small amount of insulin continuously (**basal insulin**) and when a meal is eaten, the pancreas rapidly secretes a large amount of insulin (**bolus**). Note **Figure 18: Normal Insulin Action.**[12] For the patient with diabetes to maintain as close to normal BG as possible, the insulin delivery needs to mimic the normal pancreatic secretion of insulin. In this chapter insulin therapy, including the types of insulin will be discussed. Self-Monitoring Blood Glucose (SMBG) is always necessary to assess action of any insulin.

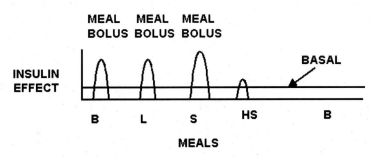

Figure 18: Normal Insulin Action

Special Insulin Therapy Tips

Special Insulin Therapy Tips to help to achieve near normal BG:

- The onset, peak action and duration of any suspended (cloudy) insulin is dependent upon adequate suspension. To insure adequate suspension of any cloudy insulin it is recommended that the vial of insulin be rolled or rocked a minimum of 20 times before each use. Failure to do this can lead to improper suspension and day to day variability in solution concentration.

- Even when refrigerated, insulin potency begins to decline 30–45 days after use despite the expiration date on the bottle. The package insert should be read to determine the duration of time an opened bottle or insulin pen can be used. Using insulin past this date can potentially lead to deterioration in BG control due to diminished potency of the insulin.

- Insulin should be stored at room temperature (>36° and < 86°)

- Mixing insulin:

  - Regular and NPH insulin can be mixed and remain stable for up to 2 weeks.

  - Regular and Lente or Regular and Ultra Lente are unstable unless immediately injected after preparation.

  - NPH and Velosulin Regular can be mixed, however they should not be mixed with Lente insulin.

  - **Glargine (Lantus) and Detemir (Levemir) CANNOT be mixed with ANY other insulin preparation!**

- Insulin pens may be used to:

  - Encourage multiple-dose insulin therapy
  - Add convenience
  - Enhance flexibility in schedule
  - Reduce insulin waste
  - Improve accuracy of dosage delivery

○ Can be used up to 10 days.

○ Humulin NPH pens can be used within 14 days.

○ Types of pre-filled pens:

  − Humalog

  − Humalog Mix 75/25

  − Humulin 70/30

  − Lantus

  − Levemir

  − Novolin 70/30

  − Novolog

  − Novolog 70/30

- **Note Figure 19: Site Rotation.**

  ○ Injections sites vary in absorption rate. The abdomen is the preferred site for inject and absorbs insulin in the most consistent fashion. The upper, outer aspects of the arm and the thigh have slower rates of absorption and more vari-

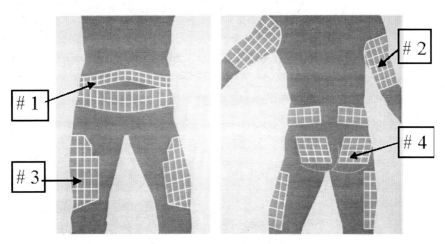

Rate of Absorption

Figure 19: Site Rotation

ability if the patient uses either extremity after injection. The buttocks are slowest absorption rate of all four sites.

○ Insulin injections need to be rotated within the site for the time of day.

○ Insulin should not be injected into the site that will be active, *i.e.* the leg before running or the arm before shoveling snow.

Action of Insulin

The summary of **Figure 20: Action of Insulin** lists the onset of action, peak action and effective duration.[6, 9]

Rapid-acting insulin is used for the **bolus** insulin. Note the action of lispro (Humalog) vs. regular insulin in **Figure 21: Biological Action of Insulin Lispro vs. Regular Insulin.**[13]

• The biological action of lispro peaks at about one hour and disappears by about 4 hours.

• In contrast, the biological action of regular insulin peaks between two and four hours after injection, with a duration of eight to ten hours.

• Because of the faster onset of lispro, the BG 2 H PC is improved.

• Because of the shorter duration of lispro, hypoglycemia (low BG) occurs less frequently later.

Therefore, the patients who benefit from lispro (Humalog), aspart (NovoLog), or glulisine (Apidra) compared with regular insulin are:

• Insulin pump users
• Older patients risk for hypoglycemia
• Surgical patients
• Patients who travel and dine out often and at erratic times
• Recurrent nocturnal and/or postprandial hypoglycemia
• Those who regularly dine late at night and snack often

ACTION OF INSULIN

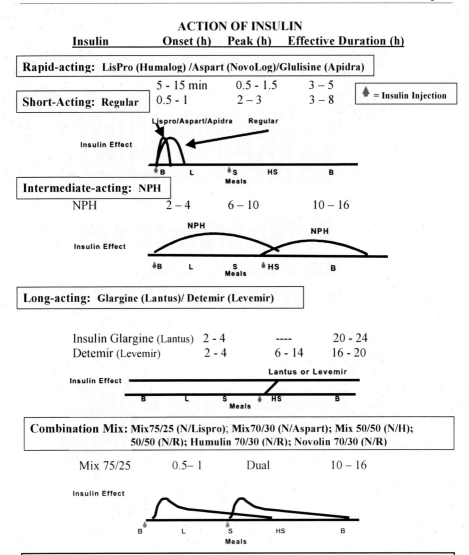

Insulin	Onset (h)	Peak (h)	Effective Duration (h)
Rapid-acting: LisPro (Humalog) /Aspart (NovoLog)/Glulisine (Apidra)			
	5 - 15 min	0.5 - 1.5	3 – 5
Short-Acting: Regular	0.5 - 1	2 – 3	3 – 8

🌲 = Insulin Injection

Intermediate-acting: NPH

NPH	2 – 4	6 – 10	10 – 16

Long-acting: Glargine (Lantus)/ Detemir (Levemir)

Insulin Glargine (Lantus)	2 - 4	----	20 - 24
Detemir (Levemir)	2 - 4	6 - 14	16 - 20

Combination Mix: Mix75/25 (N/Lispro); Mix70/30 (N/Aspart); Mix 50/50 (N/H); 50/50 (N/R); Humulin 70/30 (N/R); Novolin 70/30 (N/R)

Mix 75/25	0.5– 1	Dual	10 – 16

Time course of action of any insulin can vary in different people, or at different times in the same person; thus, time periods indicated here should be considered general guidelines only. SMBG before meals, two hours after meals, bedtime, and during the night is necessary to determine the action of insulin for each individual patient.

Figure 20: Action of Insulin

41

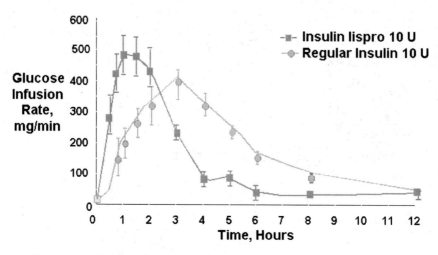

Figure 21: Biological Action of Insulin Lispro vs. Regular Insulin

- Children with unpredictable eating habits
- Dieters and erratic eaters
- Patients who exercise regularly
- Patients with gastroparesis
- Patients with type 2 diabetes who need insulin
- Patients with insulin allergy
- Patients with insulin resistance[14]

Timing of the insulin injection is important. (Note table below.) Regular insulin should usually be taken about 15 to 30 minutes prior to eating. If the BG is >200, regular insulin should be taken 60 minutes or one hour prior to eating. This is difficult for most people!

Timing of insulin injection according to BG:		
BG	Humalog/NovoLog	Regular
<50	* Meal complete	* Meal complete
50–80	* At meal time	* At meal time
80–120	* 5 min ac	* 15 min ac
120–180	* 10 min ac	* 30 min ac
>180	* 15 min ac	* 45 min ac
>200	* 20 min ac	* 60 min ac

Intermediate-acting insulin can be used for split-mixed insulin regimens that will be discussed in Chapter 6. Note **Figure 20: Action of Insulin.**

Basal insulin is achieved with **Long-acting Ultralente or Lantus.** (Note **Figure 20: Action of Insulin**). Ultralente may not last the entire twenty-four hours and may have a slight peak effect. Studies are being done to determine if Lantus may peak in about twelve hours for some patients. Therefore, care needs to be taken to prevent hypoglycemia. Also, Lantus may not actually last twenty-four hours; therefore, careful SMBG needs to be done.

Combination insulin: Note **Figure 20: Action of Insulin.**
Pros:

- Combination insulin is convenient and possibly more accurate for type 2 patients because the two types of insulin are already mixed in the vial or insulin pen.

Cons:

- The disadvantage is that the dosage cannot be changed, *i.e.* if the BG is elevated, an increased amount of rapid acting insulin cannot be given without also increasing the intermediate acting insulin.

Types:

- Humalog Mix 75/25: 75% NPH / 25% Lispro (Humalog) (Eli Lilly)
- Novolog Mix 70/30: 70% NPH / 30% Aspart (NovoLog) (Novo Nordisk)
- Novolin 70/30: 70% NPH / 30% Regular (Novo Nordisk)
- Humulin 70/30: 70% NPH / 30% Regular (Eli Lilly)
- Humalog 50/50: 50% NPH / 50% Lispro (Humalog) (Lilly)
- Humulin 50/50: 50% NPH/50% Regular (Lilly)

Insulin Therapy: Regimens

6

Insulin Regimens

Figure 22: Insulin Regimens describes the various insulin regimens which may be used to assist patients with diabetes to reach the clinical target goals of BG and A_{1c}. Reaching these goals can prevent the complications of type 1 and type 2 diabetes. These goals are listed on **Figure 13: Clinical Target Goals for Diabetes.**

The insulin regimens are listed from the simplest (2 injections/day) regimen to the more challenging regimen for the Continuous Subcutaneous Insulin Infusion (CSII) pump therapy. The regimen for combination insulin mix for type 2 is listed last. This **Figure 22: Insulin Regimens** may be used as an educational hand-out to inform diabetes patients about the action of the insulin for the various insulin regimens. The pros and cons of each regimen should be discussed with the diabetes patient to achieve adherence to the regimen and teach self-management skills.

Split-Mixed (Breakfast/Dinner)

Split-Mixed (breakfast/dinner) is two injections of NPH with lispro (Humalog), aspart (NovoLog), or glulisine (Apidra) before breakfast and dinner.

45

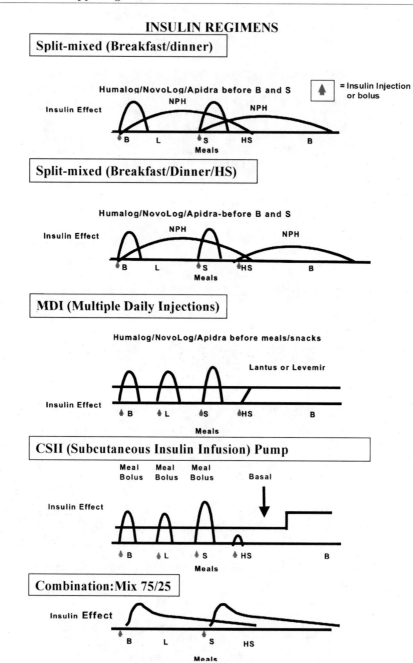

Figure 22: Insulin Regimens

Pros:

- Improves breakfast and dinner SMBG 2 H PC
- Provides basal coverage throughout the day
- Allows for fine-tuning of insulin dosages

Cons:

- Inconvenient
- Compliance issue
- Questionable accuracy of free-mixing
- If pen therapy is used, 2 injections of each type of insulin twice a day are required

How to transfer:

- Unit for unit, with rapid-acting insulin:NPH ratio of about 1:2
- $^2/_3$ of Total Daily Dose (TDD) of insulin in AM: *i.e.:* 13 U lispro, aspart, or Regular, 27 U NPH at breakfast
- $^1/_3$ of TDD of insulin before dinner: *i.e.:* 6 U lispro, aspart, or Regular, 13 U NPH at dinner

Split-Mixed (Breakfast/Dinner/Bedtime)

Split-Mixed (breakfast/dinner/HS-bedtime) is three injections: NPH with lispro, aspart, or Regular before breakfast, lispro, aspart, or Regular before dinner, and NPH at bedtime.

Pros:

- Coverage for the Dawn Phenomenon with NPH taken at HS (bedtime), not dinner
- Reduces nocturnal hypoglycemia
- FPG improved
- Breakfast & dinner SMBG 2 H PC improved

- Provides basal coverage throughout the day
- Allows for fine-tuning of insulin dosages

Cons:
- Inconvenient
- Possible compliance issue for 3 injections/day
- Questionable accuracy of free-mixing

How to transfer:
- Unit for unit, with lispro:NPH ratio of about 1:2
- $^2/_3$ of TDD (Total Daily Dose) of insulin in AM: *i.e.:* 13 U lispro, aspart, or Regular, 27 U NPH at breakfast
- $^1/_3$ of TDD of insulin before dinner/HS: *i.e.:* 6 U lispro, aspart, or Regular at dinner 13 U NPH at HS

Multiple Daily Injections (MDI)

Multiple Daily Injections (MDI) of insulin mimics the normal pancreas. MDI has been shown to provide near normal BG results for type 1 and type 2 patients.[1, 9, 12] The patient will be taking four injections.

- Basal insulin is provided with long-acting Glargine (Lantus®) or Detemir (Levemir®) insulin. This insulin maintains a basal amount of insulin. It can be given at HS, before breakfast, or bid. The basal insulin is usually about 40–50% of the TDD for twenty-four hours. Some clinicians use long-acting insulin for type 2 patients with SU and/or TZD and/or Metformin therapy.
- Bolus insulin is provided with rapid insulin: Lispro (Humalog® by Lilly), aspart (Novolog® by Novo Nordisk) or glulisine (Apidra®). The bolus for the meal is injected when and if the meal is eaten for the amount of food eaten. Therefore, the patient needs to learn to do CHO counting to calculate the amount of insulin needed for the amount of food eaten. Calculations for insulin will be discussed later in Chapter 7.

Pros:
- SMBG, especially 2 H PC improved
- Provides basal coverage throughout the day
- Allows for fine-tuning of insulin dosages
- Reduces nocturnal hypoglycemia
- Flexibility for improved lifestyle: give bolus when, and if, food is eaten for the amount of food eaten
- A_{1c} results improved

Cons:
- Four or more injections/day
- CHO counting is necessary
- Sensitivity Factor/Correction Formula (CF) is necessary
- Inconvenient
- Compliance issue with multiple injections
- Questionable accuracy of free-mixing

How to transfer:
- Lantus 40–50% of TDD/24 hours (see Chapter 7)
- Bolus calculated from Insulin: CHO ratio (see Chapter 7)
- CF calculated (see Chapter 7)

Continuous Subcutaneous Insulin Infusion (CSII) Pump

Continuous Subcutaneous Insulin Infusion (CSII) Pump mimics the normal pancreas and has been shown to provide near normal BG results for type 1 and type 2 patients.[9, 15, 16] The insulin pump is worn continuously with a Teflon needle inserted into the abdomen. The needle is changed every two to four days by the patient. Extensive diabetes education of self-management skills is necessary with a diabetes nurse educator and dietitian diabetes educator. Rapid-acting insulin (Humalog, NovoLog, or Apidra)) only is used in the insulin pump.

- Basal insulin is provided with a continuous delivery of small amounts of rapid-acting insulin only. The basal insulin is programmed into the pump according to the individual's need. Different basal rates of insulin can be programmed throughout the day, *i.e.* a higher basal rate during the night to cover the Dawn Phenomenon.

- Bolus insulin is taken when the patient is ready for a meal. He/she programs the pump for the amount of insulin needed for the amount of food at the meal.

Pros:[15, 16]

- Improved blood glucose control
- Prevention and delay of the progression of complications[1]
- Precise dosage delivery[1, 5, 9]
- Management of Dawn Phenomenon
- Improved BG control during exercise
- Decreased hypoglycemia
- Improved gastroparesis management
- Improved BG control for pre-conception and pregnancy
- Increased flexibility in lifestyle

Pros during pregnancy:[17]

- Mimics normal physiology
- Decreases glucose excursions
- Reduces hypoglycemia
- Reduces risk of DKA
- Provides individualization of insulin regimen
- Improves management of morning sickness
- Increases lifestyle flexibility

Pros for type 2 patients:[18]

- Decreases insulin resistance

- Reduces glucose toxicity
- Restores sensitivity to oral medications and diet

Cons:

- Learning curve
- Risk of DKA (with only rapid-acting insulin in pump)
- Possible weight gain
- Frequent monitoring required
- Potential site infections
- Inconvenience in wearing pump
- Education and follow-up required
- Cost

Combination Insulin

Combination Insulin:

Types:

- Humalog Mix 75/25: 75% NPH/25% Lispro (Humalog) (Eli Lilly)
- Novolog Mix 70/30: 70% NPH/30% Aspart (NovoLog) (Novo Nordisk)
- Novolin 70/30: 70% NPH/30% Regular (Novo Nordisk)
- Humulin 70/30: 70% NPH/30% Regular (Eli Lilly)
- Humalog 50/50: 50% NPH/50% Lispro (Humalog) (Lilly)
- Humulin 50/50: 50% NPH/50% Regular (Lilly)

Pros:

- Convenient pre-mix simple dosing, especially for type 2 patients
- Basal coverage provided throughout the day
- Breakfast and dinner SMBG 2 H PC improved

Cons:

- Cannot fine-tune
- Lispro component, if taken too long before eating, can cause hypoglycemia

How to transfer:

- 2/3 TDD in AM: *i.e.* 40 U at breakfast
- 1/3 TDD at dinner: *i.e.* 20 U at dinner

New Developments:

Exubera® is an inhaled insulin system. The peak of action is 49 minutes and is to be used prior to meals with NPH, Lantus, or Levemir insulin injected. Lung function needs to be measured initially, then every six to twelve months. Exubera should not be used for patients with asthma, bronchitis, emphysema or having a history of smoking within the last six months. Exubera was taken off the market October, 2007, however, other manufacturers are planning an inhaled insulin as well.

Insulin Therapy: Calculating Dosage

7

Calculating Insulin Dosage

To start insulin therapy, the following calculations need to be done:

- Total Daily Dose (TDD)
- Basal Rate
- Bolus
- Insulin Sensitivity Factor/Correction Formula
- Unused Insulin Rule
- Target Goal BG (See Chapter 3)

Total Daily Dose

TDD is the total amount of all of the insulin for the 24 hour period. If a patient who weighs 260 pounds and is receiving Humalog 13 U with NPH 27 U at breakfast, 6 U of Humalog at dinner, and 13 U of NPH at bedtime, the total amount (TDD) would be 59 Units. To calculate kilograms, divide the weight in pounds by 2.2.

To calculate this patient's Units/kg:
Units TDD ÷ kg = _____ U/kg/24 hours

Example:
260 ÷ 2.2 = 118 kg
TDD of 59 Units ÷ 118 = 0.5 U/kg/24 hours.

The TDD calculation assists in determining if the patient is receiving an appropriate amount of insulin in 24 hours. For a non-pregnant adult the dose should be approximately 0.5–0.7 U/kg.

The TDD calculation is also dependent upon the patient's body mass measured in kilograms.

TDD (Total Daily Dose)/24 hours[19, 20]	
	U/kg body weight
• Non-pregnancy	0.5–0.7
• Honeymoon	0.4
• Elderly	0.3
During pregnancy the insulin requirements increase as discussed earlier:[17]	
Pregnancy:	U/kg body weight
• Weeks 2–16	0.7
• Weeks 16–26	0.8
• Weeks 26–36	0.9
• Weeks 36–40 +	1.0
• Obese (>150% desirable body weight)	1.5–2.0

Examples: (non-pregnant adults)	
Patient A weighs 130 pounds.	Patient B weighs 210 pounds.
130 lbs = 59kg × 0.5 =	210 lbs = 95.5kg × 0.5 =
29.5U TDD/24 hrs	47.8U TDD/24 hrs

- These formulas are a method for determining if the patient is getting the approximately correct amount of insulin. This needs to be individualized and titrated by the patient doing SMBG AC, 2 H PC, HS, and during the night.
- The lower amount (0.5 U/kg/24 hrs) is used and then the dosage is titrated.
- Too much insulin will cause hypoglycemia, hunger and result in weight gain.
- Insufficient insulin will cause hyperglycemia and result in the complications of diabetes.
- The honeymoon phase may or may not occur with the newly diagnosed type 1 patient, and less insulin may be needed for a period of time. Each patient is different!

Basal Dose of Insulin

In MDI and CSII therapies it is necessary to calculate the amount of basal insulin. The **basal** dose of insulin (long-acting insulin) should be 40–50% of TDD.[15, 16, 19, 20] The basal dose would utilize Lantus for MDI or the basal rate insulin for CSII (Continuous Subcutaneous Insulin Infusion) pump therapy.

Example:	Example:
Patient A	Patient B
29.5U (TDD) × 0.4 (40%) = 11.8U	47.8U (TDD) × 0.4 (40%) = 19U
Round 11.8U off to 12U. This would be the amount of Lantus or Levemir for MDI or the basal total for CSII	This would be the amount of Lantus or Levemir for MDI or the basal total for CSII

To determine the basal rate for CSII, the basal total is divided by 24 hours of the day:

Example:	Example:
Patient A	Patient B
11.8 ÷ 24 hours = .49 or 0.5 U/hour The basal rate for the CSII pump would then be set at 0.5U/hour	19 ÷ 24 hours = 0.79 or 0.8 U/hour The basal rate for the CSII pump would then be set at 0.8U/hour

- These formulas provide a method for determining the patient dosage. This needs to be individualized and titrated by the patient doing SMBG AC, 2 H PC, HS, and during the night.
- The lower amount (40%) is used to calculate the basal amount of insulin and then the dosage is titrated.

Multiple Basal Rate Calculations for CSII

The basal rate is programmed into the CSII pump. When starting pump therapy one continuous basal rate may be set, *i.e.* Patient A would have 0.5U/hour set in the pump. Frequently, multiple basal rates are needed and programmed. More insulin is usually needed for the Dawn Phenomenon. The following formulas can be used to calculate multiple basal rates:

- Rate 1 (starts 12 midnight-sleeping): $^1/_2$ of Rate 3
- Rate 2 (Dawn Phenomenon): 1.5 × Rate 3
- Rate 3* (daytime): 40–50% TDD
- Rate 4 (sleeping): $^1/_2$ of Rate 3 (same as Rate 1)[17]

When calculating multiple basal rates for CSII:

- The programming begins at midnight.
- *Rate 3 (daytime rate) is calculated and usually started at first for the entire twenty-four hours.
- Increasing or decreasing adjustments of the basal rate are titrated according to SMBG results.

Meal Bolus

The **Meal Bolus** amount (rapid-acting insulin) is approximately 50–60% of TDD. The meal bolus is the rapid-acting insulin (Humalog, NovoLog, or Apidra) taken at meal time when, and if, food is eaten for the amount of food that is eaten. This method is used for both MDI and CSII:[15, 16, 17, 21]

Calculating Meal Bolus:

- **500 Rule: for rapid-acting insulin**
  500 ÷ TDD = 1 U insulin to ___ grams (g) CHO

- **450 Rule: for regular**
  450 ÷ TDD = 1 U insulin to ___ g CHO

The amount of meal bolus may need to be larger for patients exhibiting insulin resistance:

- Teens
- Patients exhibiting BG results of the Dawn Phenomenon (breakfast)
- Type 2

Example:	Example:
Patient A	Patient B
500 ÷ 29.5 (TDD) = 16.7 Patient A would use 1U of rapid-acting insuling for 16.7 (round off to 15–17) g CHO	500 ÷ 47.8 (TDD) = 10.5 Patient B would use 1U of rapid-acting insulin for 10.5 (round off to 10–11) g CHO

- These formulas are a method for determining the patient's meal bolus dosage. This needs to be individualized and titrated by the patient doing SMBG especially the 2 H PC.
- Instruction of CHO counting by a dietitian diabetes educator is crucial.
- Various CHO counting books are available to assist the patient to count CHO accurately.

Insulin Sensitivity Factor/Correction Formula

Insulin Sensitivity Factor/Correction Formula[15, 16, 20] determines how the patient responds to 1 unit (U) of insulin and can be used for hyperglycemia, hypoglycemia, and sick day management. This was formerly called the sliding scale of insulin.

Insulin Sensitivity Factor

- 1800 Rule: For rapid-acting insulin
  1800 ÷ TDD = 1 U ↓ BG ___ mg/dL

- 1500 Rule: For regular
  1500 ÷ TDD = 1 U ↓ BG ___ mg/dL

Example:	Example:
Patient A	Patient B

1800 ÷ 29.5 (TDD)
  = 61 mg/dL
Patient A would take 1U of rapid-acting insulin to lower the BG 61 mg/dL.
	1800 ÷ 47.8 (TDD)
	  = 37.7 mg/dL
	Patient B would take 1U of rapid-acting insulin to lower the BG 38 mg/dL (round off 37.7 to 38).

- The correction formula is:
  Current BG minus target BG = amount to correct ÷ insulin sensitivity factor

Examples:

Patient A has a current BG of 170mg/dL

- 170mg/dL – 110mg/dL (average target of 90–130mg/dL) = 60mg/dL ÷ 61 (sensitivity factor) = 1 U of rapid-acting insulin.
- Patient A would take 1 U of rapid-acting insulin to bring the BG down to target or add Humalog, NovoLog, or Apidra 1 U to the meal bolus to bring the BG down to target.

Patient A has a current BG of 50 mg/dL

- 50mg/dL – 110 mg/dL = –60mg/dL ÷ 61 = –1 U of rapid-acting insulin.
- Patient A would subtract 1 U of Humalog, NovoLog,or Apidra from the meal bolus.

- Total bolus = meal bolus +/– correction formula amount
- These formulas are a method for assessing the patient dosage. This needs to be individualized and titrated by the patient doing SMBG AC, 2 H PC, HS, and during the night.

Unused Insulin Rule

The **unused insulin rule** tells how many units of insulin remain from the previous bolus. Hypoglycemia can occur from taking a correction factor bolus after any other bolus has been given because some of the insulin from the previous bolus still remains.[16]

- **Humalog or NovoLog** is depleted in approx. 3–4 hrs

  Decrease bolus 30% each hour:

  1st hour = 70% remaining

  2nd hour = 40% remaining

  3rd hour = 10% remaining

  4th hour = 0 remaining

- **Regular** is depleted in approx. 5 hrs

  Decrease bolus 20% each hour:

  1st hour = 80% remaining

  2nd hour = 60% remaining

  3rd hour = 40% remaining

  4th hour = 20% remaining

  5th hour = 0 remaining

Example:

Patient A has current BG 2 H PC of 300mg/dL

- 300mg/dL – 160 (target BG for 2 H PC) = 140mg/dL ÷ 61 (sensitivity factor) = Humalog or NovoLog 2.3U × 0.4 (40% unused insulin) = 0.9U (round off 0.9U to 1U)
- Therefore, Patient A would only take 1U of Humalog or NovoLog 2 H PC for the 300mg/dL BG.

- These formulas are a method for determining the patient dosage. This needs to be individualized and titrated by the patient doing SMBG AC, 2 H PC, HS, and during the night.

Amylin (pramlintide acetate-Symlin®)

The dosing and titration guide for Amylin (Symlin®) injections used for Type 1 patients are as follows: (*See* **Chapter 4** for dosing for Type 2 patients)

- Begin Symlin at a dose of 2.5 units (15μ)
- Reduce mealtime insulin by 50%
- Inject immediately prior to meals of at least 250 calories or 30 grams of CHO
- Increase dose by 2.5-unit increments up to 10 units (60μ) as tolerated when there has been no nausea for 3 or more days
- If nausea persists at the 7.5 unit (45μ) or 10 unit (60μ) doses, reduce dose to 5 units (30μ)

These recommendations are a guide for the medical management of the patient with type 1 or 2 diabetes and are meant only as an estimated initiation guide that should be modified by patient experience and clinical judgment. The process usually requires at least four weeks with significant patient education (utilizing a diabetes nurse educator and dietitian diabetes educator) and coaching of self-management skills.

Troubleshooting Blood Glucose Control 8

Balancing Blood Glucose Control

Management of diabetes is a balancing act of making careful assessments of BG results to achieve target BG and A_{1c}. A balance of the amount of food intake, activity, and diabetes medication and/or insulin or CSII pump dosage needs to be achieved. Note **Figure 23: Balancing Act.** Thorough evaluation of SMBG results will determine the possible causes for the hyperglycemia or hypoglycemia.

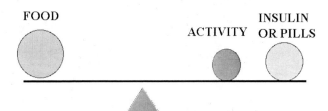

FOOD   INSULIN
ACTIVITY   OR PILLS

Figure 23: Balancing Act

If the target BG and A_{1c} is not reached, use **Figure 24: Troubleshooting Guide** to assess the need for changes in the diabetes management. Food intake, activity, medication and/or insulin, SMBG, and other factors need to be considered.

TROUBLESHOOTING GUIDE

Possible causes for *high* blood glucose

Food intake:
>Unplanned increase in amount of food
>Meal bolus insufficient or omitted (CHO:insulin ratio incorrect)
>Improper oral medications or insulin bolus at time of meal
>Increased fat or protein meal
>Snacking; long meal (holiday)
>Slowly absorbed foods (high fiber)
>Over treating hypoglycemia
>Gastroparesis

Activity:
>Lack of or reduced activity
>>240 BG <u>WITH</u> ketones before exercise—may cause higher BG
>>300 BG without ketones—may cause higher BG
>CSII: over use of temporary basal rate or suspend for activity

Oral Medication (type 2):
>Omitted or insufficient amount (need to increase to maximum dose)
>Need addition of combination of oral medications
>Beta cell failure (normal occurrence)—need to begin insulin

Insulin:
>Omitted or insufficient amount of insulin (basal or bolus)
>Cloudy or clumpy
>Expired
>Exposed to temperature extremes
>Improper bolus timing with meal
>Correction Factor insufficient/incorrect
>Injection site—hypertrophy, nodule

SMBG (Self-Monitoring Blood Glucose):
>Insufficient number of SMBG tests
>Questionable accuracy of SMBG
>Not recording SMBG
>Not checking 3AM BG
>Somogyi rebound (elevated BG after low BG)
>Dawn phenomenon (need to check during the night)

Other factors:
>Weight increase
>Emotional stress
>Illness, infection, fever
>Menses, menopause
>Growth spurts

Figure 24: Troubleshooting Guide

Medication, *i.e.* steroids, anti-depressives, HCTZ, etc.
CSII (Continuous Subcutaneous Insulin Infusion Pump):
Infusion site: inflamed, red, irritated, nodule
Infusion set: not primed (air in tubing)
Insulin leakage at site
Needle dislodged or cannula kinked
Blood in infusion set
Set inserted at HS
Cannula bolus omitted
Insufficient basal rate
Basal rate programmed incorrectly
Pump in SUSPEND
Pump malfunction
Occlusion alarm
Clock time incorrect
Low or dead battery

CSII PUMP THERAPY: WHEN IN DOUBT, CHANGE IT OUT!
For unaccounted blood glucose ≥ 240 mg/dL two times in a row, change the pump cartridge and infusion set; check ketones. Take fast acting insulin by syringe as directed by your physician or healthcare professional.

Possible causes for *low* blood glucose

Food intake:
Too much bolus; CHO:insulin ratio incorrect
Delayed, omitted, or lost meal
Less Food eaten than planned
Gastroparesis: BG low when eating meal
Improper timing of bolus (too early)
Alcohol consumption
Weight loss
Activity:
Long duration or unplanned activity (*i.e.* shopping, biking, etc.)
(See CHO replacement for Exercise chart)
Extended or intensive activity (can cause low BG 24–36 hrs later)
Did not decrease amount of oral medication or insulin
SMBG:
Insufficient number of SMBG tests
Questionable accuracy of SMBG
Not recording SMBG
BG unchecked during night

Figure 24: Troubleshooting Guide (Continued)

History of unconscious or severe low BG
Hypoglycemia unawareness (no symptoms)
Oral medication or Insulin:
 Too much oral medication or insulin (basal or bolus)
 Improper timing of oral medication or insulin
 Frequent bolus (observe unused insulin rule)
CSII Pump:
 Basal rate programmed incorrectly
 Clock time incorrect
 Insulin bolus: CHO ratio incorrect

Rule of 15 for treating low BG

- Consume 15 grams of quick-acting carbohydrate.
  Wait 15 minutes; recheck blood glucose.
  If glucose level is <60 mg/dl, repeat above.
- Carry quick-acting CHO
- Check BG before driving (needs to be >100 mg/dL)
- Wear Medic Alert
- Glucagon* for severe hypoglycemia from insulin
  *(To be given by significant other)

CHO Replacement for Exercise
(Long duration or unplanned exercise)

INTENSITY	DURATION (min)	CHO	FREQUENCY
Mild-to-mod	<30	may not need	---
Moderate	30–60	15 g	each hr
High	60+	30–50 g	each hr

Figure 24: Troubleshooting Guide (Continued)

Troubleshooting Guide: High BG Results

This guide lists possible causes for *high* **BG** (hyperglycemia) results. It is necessary to check SMBG 2 hours after meals (BG 2 H PC). If the meal bolus (rapid-acting insulin) or amount of oral medication is insufficient, the BG 2 H PC will be elevated as shown in **Figure 25: Insufficient Meal Bolus.**

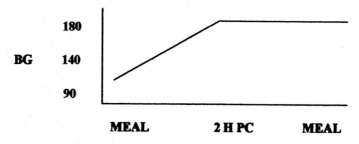

Figure 25: Insufficient Meal Bolus

Figure 26: Insufficient Basal Insulin shows a normal BG 2 H PC, however the BG AC (before the next meal) is elevated. This might indicate that the basal amount of oral medication (TZD, Biguanide) or insulin (Lantus, Ultralente, NPH, or CSII basal rate) is insufficient.

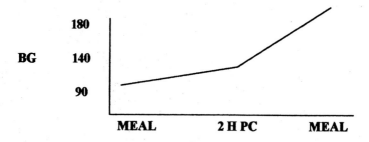

Figure 26: Insufficient Basal Insulin

SMBG Check During the Night

The following figures show all of the possibilities that can occur during the night time hours. Studies have shown that patients with diabetes may not be aware of hypoglycemia occurring during the night. Therefore, SMBG must be checked at bedtime (HS), during the night, and the next morning (FPG [Fasting Plasma Glucose]).

Figure 27: Insufficient Insulin shows an elevation of BG during the night. This indicates insufficient insulin taken for HS snack, or not enough oral medication or basal insulin.

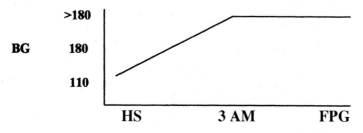

Figure 27: Insufficient Insulin

Figure 28: Insufficient Basal Insulin shows a continual elevation of BG during the night. This indicates insufficient oral medication or basal insulin.

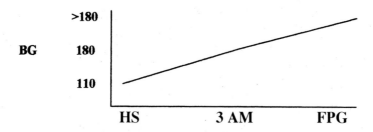

Figure 28: Insufficient Basal Insulin

Figure 29: Dawn Phenomenon shows the BG normal during the first part of the night, then elevates. This indicates the dawn phenomenon discussed in Chapter 1 (**Figure 2: Hormones That Affect BG** and **Figure 3: Dawn Phenomenon**).

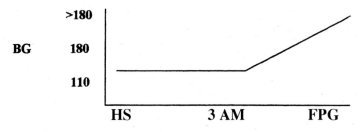

Figure 29: Dawn Phenomenon

Figure 30: Too Much Insulin Causing Somogyi Rebound shows a low BG during the night. This indicates too much bolus insulin or oral medication was taken for HS snack or too much basal insulin. Somogyi is post-hypoglycemic hyperglycemia, *i.e.* BG results are elevated after a low BG. The low BG is a "stress" to the system stimulating the adrenal gland to secrete adrenaline causing the liver to give off the glycogen (sugar) stores, therefore causing an elevated BG. This can also occur during the daytime hours.

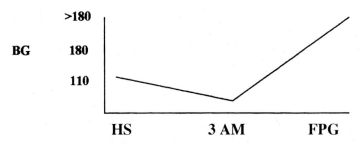

Figure 30: Too Much Insulin Causing Somogyi Rebound

Figure 31: Too Much Insulin shows a low BG during the night and in the morning hours. This indicates too much oral medication or bolus insulin taken for HS snack or too much basal insulin. Hypoglycemia can also occur 24 hours after strenuous exercise.

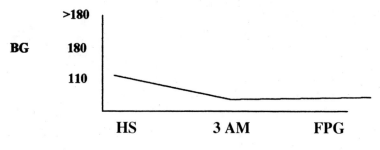

Figure 31: Too Much Insulin

Sick days can also alter target BG results. **Figure 32: Sick Day Guidelines** is a sample of a hand-out for type 1 or type 2 or CSII users.

SICK DAY GUIDELINES

During periods of short-term illness, it may be more difficult to maintain good control of your diabetes. Examples of minor illness are: dental surgery, colds, nausea/vomiting, sore throat, mild infections, diarrhea, and fever.

CALL YOUR HEALTH CARE PROFESSIONAL IF:

❖ Illness continues without improvement
❖ Temperature >100 degrees F
❖ Vomiting or diarrhea continues longer than 4 hours
❖ Moderate to large amount of ketones are present in the urine
❖ Blood sugar levels continue to run less than 60 mg/dL, or above 240 mg/dL (above 130 mg/dL during pregnancy) after taking extra insulin doses as pre-arranged with your physician.
❖ Signs of ketoacidosis, dehydration or other serious problems such as increased drowsiness, abdominal or chest pain, difficulty breathing, fruity odor to breath, dry cracked lips, mouth or tongue are present
❖ Any illness that lasts more than 24 hours
❖ Illness continues without improvement
❖ There is any uncertainty about what you need to do to take care of yourself

---

Medication: **Never omit your medication or insulin!** If you are ill and cannot eat, your need for insulin continues and may also increase. You may need extra insulin according to your sensitivity factor or supplemental insulin scale.

Blood/Urine Testing:
➢ Test blood sugar at least before your usual meal time and every 2-4 hours if indicated.
➢ Test your urine for ketones at least 4 times per day.

Fluids/Diet:
➢ Start fluids 1 or 2 hours after any vomiting and drink the fluids slowly.
➢ Consume 10-15 grams of carbohydrate every 1-2 hours.
➢ If blood glucose >250mg/dL: **Drink:** water, teas with no sugar, instant broth, diet drinks
Eat: ice chips, sugar-free ice popsicles, sugar-free gelatin
➢ If blood glucose <250mg/dL: **Drink:** fruit juice, ginger ale, or regular soda **OR**
Eat: glucose tablets, regular ice popsicles, regular sugar gelatin, soups

---

Figure 32 Sick Day Guidelines

Troubleshooting Guide: Low BG Results

Figure 24: Troubleshooting Guide lists possible causes and also the treatment for low BG (hypoglycemia) results.

Figure 33: Too Much Meal Bolus shows the necessity of checking SMBG 2 H PC. If the meal bolus (rapid-acting insulin) or amount of oral medication is too high, the 2 H PC BG will be lower than the target BG.

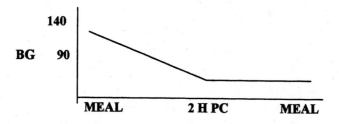

Figure 33: Too Much Meal Bolus

Figure 34: Too Much Meal Bolus Causing Somogyi Rebound shows an elevated BG at the next meal time after a low BG 2 H PC. This is the Somogyi effect described earlier.

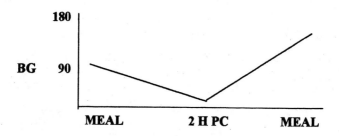

Figure 34: Too Much Meal Bolus Causing Somogyi Rebound

Figure 35: Too Much Basal Insulin shows a normal BG 2 H PC, however the C (before the next meal) is low. This might indicate that the basal amount of oral medication (TZD, Biguanide) or insulin (Lantus, Ultralente, NPH, or CSII basal rate) is too high.

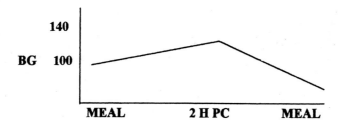

Figure 35: Too Much Basal Insulin

In Summary: Health Care Professionals today are working with increasing numbers of diabetes patients. The incidence of type 2 diabetes is in epidemic proportions due to obesity and sedentary lifestyles leading to insulin resistance. The devastating complications of diabetes remain one of the leading causes of death. By utilizing oral medication and insulin to mimic the normal pancreatic function and reaching target BG and A_{1c} these complications can be prevented, and patients with diabetes can improve their quality of life. Since Health Care Professionals are working with diabetes patients to make changes in their medical management, it is important to remember ". . . changes in attitudes, beliefs, and understandings tend to follow rather than precede changes in behavior."(from M. Fullan, 1985).

Bibliography for Footnotes

1   Diabetes Control and Complications Trail Research Group: The Effect of Intensive Treatment of Diabetes on the Development and Progression of Long-Term Complications in Insulin-Dependent Diabetes Mellitus. *N Engl J of Med:* 329;977–986, 1993.

2   UK Prospective Diabetes Study Group: Intensive Blood-Glucose Control with Sulfonylureas or Insulin Compared with Conventional Treatment and Risk of Complications in Patients with Type 2 Diabetes (UKPDS 33). *Lancet:* 352:837–853, 1998.

3   Bobak, et al: The Nurse and the Family. *Maternity and Gynecologic Care:* 783, 1989.

4   Bastyr III, et al: Therapy Focused on Lowering Postprandial Glucose, Not Fasting Glucose, May Be Superior for Lowering A_{1c}. *Diabetes Care:* 23:1236–1241, 2000.

5   Pfeifer, MA, et al: *Am J Med:* 70–579, 1981.

6   American Diabetes Association: Clinical Practice Recommendations 2008. *Diabetes Care:* 26(Suppl 1):S1–S156, 2008.

7   Kaufman, et al: *Contemporary Pediatrics:* 16:112, 1999.

8   Diabetes Nutrition Practice Guidelines Pocket Guide: *A Companion Resource to the American Dietetic Association MNT Evidence Based Guides for Practice,* 2002.

9   Franz, MJ, et al: *A Core Curriculum for Diabetes Education*, 4th ed: Diabetes and Complications, Diabetes Management Therapies, Diabetes in the Life Cycle and Research: Chicago, IL: American Association of Diabetes Educators, 2001.

10 Nathan, DM, et al: Management of Hyperglycemia in Type 2 Diabetes: A Consensus Algorithm for the Initiation and Adjustment of Therapy. *Diabetes Care 29*: 1963–1972, 2006

11 Riddle, M; Rosenstock, J; HOE.901/4002 Study Group: *Diabetes.* 51(suppl 2):A113. Abstract 457-P, 2002.

12 Schade, Skyler, Santiago, Rizza: Intensive Insulin Therapy: *Excerpta Medica:* p. 131, 1983.

13 Howey, DC; et al, *Diabetes:* 43:396–402, 1994.

14 Meece, Jerry and Campbell, R. Keith, "Insulin Lispro Update," *The Diabetes Educator:* March/April, p. 269–277, 2002.

15 Bolderman, K: *Putting Your Patients on the Pump:* Alexandria, VA, American Diabetes Association, 1998.

16 Walsh, PA; Roberts, R: *Pumping Insulin:* 3rd ed. San Diego, Calif: Torrey Pines Press, 2000.

17 Jornsay, DL: CSII Therapy During Pregnancy. *Diabetes Spectrum:* 11: 26–32, 1998.

18 Ilkova, et al: *Diabetes Care:* Vol 20: p. 1353, 1997.

19 American Diabetes Association: *Intensive Diabetes Management.* 2nd ed. Alexandria, VA: ADA, 1998.

20 Davidson, P; Bode, BW: *The Insulin Pump Therapy Book: Insights From the Experts.* Sylmar, Calif: MiniMed Technologies; 49–56, 65–68, 85–93, 1995.

21 Brackenridge, BP: Carbohydrate Gram Counting. *Practical Diabetology:* 11(3):22–28, 1992.

Resources

American Association of Clinical Endocrinologists, Medical Guidelines for Clinical Practice for the Management of Diabetes Mellitus. www.aace.com/pub/pdf/guidelines/DMGuidelines 2007.pdf.

American Association of Diabetes Educators: *The Art and Science of Diabetes Self-Management Education: A Desk Reference for Healthcare Professionals:* A Core Knowledge Publication, Chicago, IL: 800 pages, 2006.

American Diabetes Association: "Evidence-Based Nutrition Principles and Recommendations for the Treatment and Prevention of Diabetes and Related Complications." *Diabetes Care* 25:S50–60, 2002.

American Diabetes Association: "Clinical Practice Recommendations," Supplement 1, 2008.

American Diabetes Association: "Complete Nurse's Guide: Diabetes Care," 470 pages, 2005.

American Diabetes Association: "Continuous Subcutaneous Insulin Infusion." *Diabetes Care* 25:S116, 2002.

American Diabetes Association: *Diabetes Medical Nutrition Therapy,* (comprehensive, practical guide to delivering nutrition advice).

American Diabetes Association: "Implications of the Diabetes Control and Complications Trial." *Diabetes Care* 25:S25–27, 2002.

American Diabetes Association: "Implications of the United Kingdom Prospective Diabetes Study." *Diabetes Care* 25:S28–32, 2002.

American Diabetes Association: "Insulin Administration." *Diabetes Care* 25:S112–115, 2002.

American Diabetes Association: *Intensive Diabetes Management.* 2nd Edition, (hands-on guide that delivers practical advice on achieving better blood glucose control) 1998. 186 pages

American Diabetes Association: *Medical Management of Pregnancy Complicated by Diabetes*, 2nd Edition. (every aspect of pregnancy and diabetes) 134 pages.

American Diabetes Association: *Medical Management of Type 1 Diabetes*, 4th Edition. (state-of-the-art instruction on all issues impacting patients with type 1 diabetes) 2004. 258 pages.

American Diabetes Association: *Medical Management of Type 2 Diabetes*, 4th Edition. (diagnosis and treatment advice about all areas of Type 2) 2004. 141 pages.

American Diabetes Association: "National Standards for Diabetes Self-Management Education." *Diabetes Care* January, 2006: S140–147.

American Diabetes Association: "Report of the Expert Committee on the Diagnosis and Classification of Diabetes Mellitus." *Diabetes Care* 25:S5–20, 2006.

American Diabetes Association: "Resource Guide 2006." *Diabetes Forecast.* (Guide for comparing features from different manufacturers for: insulin, syringes, jet injectors, insulin pumps, injection aids, aids for visually impaired, test strips, blood glucose monitors and data-management systems, finger-sticking supplies, medical ID's, and more.)

American Diabetes Association: "Standards of Medical Care for Patients with Diabetes Mellitus." *Diabetes Care* 25:S33–49, 2006.

American Diabetes Association: *The Health Professional's Guide to Diabetes and Exercise*, (comprehensive guide how to prescribe exercise therapy) 346 pages.

American Diabetes Association: *Therapy for Diabetes Mellitus and Related Disorders*, 4th Edition. (reference guide for management of patients with diabetes) 2004. 543 pages.

Bode, BW; Steed, RD; Davidson, PC: Reduction in severe hypoglycemia with long-term continuous subcutaneous insulin infusion. *Diabetes Care* 22 (Supp 1) (Reprint), 1999.

Bolderman, Karen: *Putting Your Patients on the Pump*. (complete information on CSII therapy) American Diabetes Association, 2002, 91 pages.

Brackenridge, BP: "Carbohydrate Gram Counting." *Practical Diabetology:* 11(3):22–28, 1992.

Campbell, KB, Braithwaite, SS. "Hospital Management of Hyperglycemia." *Clinical Diabetes* 22:81–87.

Clement, S, et al, "Management of Diabetes and Hyperglycemia in Hospitals," *Diabetes Care 27*, No 2, February, 2004, p. 558.

Diabetes Control and Complications Trial Research Group: The Effect of Intensive Treatment of Diabetes on the Development and Progression of Long-Term Complications in Insulin-Dependent Diabetes Mellitus, *N Engl J Med* 329:977–986, 1993.

Diabetes Prevention Research Group: Reduction in the evidence of type 2 diabetes with life-style intervention or metformin, *N Engl J Med* 346: 393–403, 2002.

Franz, M; Kulkarni, K; Polonsky, W; Yarborough, P; Zamudio, eds.: *A Core Curriculum for Health Professionals: Diabetes Management Therapies, Diabetes Education and Program Management, Diabetes and Complications, Diabetes in the Life Cycle and Research*, 4th Edition, (American Association Diabetes Educators) 2001.

Hirsch, et al: "Intensive Insulin Therapy Treatment of Type I Diabetes." *Diabetes Care* 13:1265–1283.

Jornsay, DL: "Continuous Subcutaneous Insulin Infusion (CSII) Therapy During Pregnancy." *Diabetes Spectrum* 11:26–32, 1998.

Nathan, DM, et al: "Management of Hyperglycemia in Type 2 Diabetes: A consensus Algorithm for the Initiation and Adjustment of Therapy." *Diabetes Care* 29: 1963–1972, 2006.

Skyler, et al: "Algorithms for Adjustment of Insulin Dosage by Patients Who Monitor Blood Glucose." *Diabetes Care* 311–318, March–April 1981.

Walsh, J; Roberts, R: *Pumping Insulin*, 4th ed. San Diego, CA: Torrey Pines Press, 2006.

Websites

American Association of Clinical Endocrinologists	www.aace.com
American Association of Diabetes Educations	www.aadenet.org (1-800-TEAM-UP4)
American Diabetes Association	www.diabetes.org (1-800-DIABETES)
ADA Clinical Practice Recommendations	http://care.diabetesjournals.org
ADA Education Recognition	www.diabetes.org /recognition
American Dietetic Association	www.eatright.org (1-800-877-1600)
American Heart Association	www.americanheart.org/diabetes (1-800-AHA-USA1)
Centers for Disease Control	www.cdc.gov/diabetes (1-877-232-3433)
Children with Diabetes	www.childrenwithdiabetes.com
Diabetes Action Research & Education Foundation	www.diabetesaction.org
Diabetes Division of the National Federation of the Blind	www.nfb.org/diabetes.htm
Diabetes Education and Research Center	www.libertynet.org/diabetes
Diabetes In Control	www.diabetesincontrol.com
Diabetes Interview	www.diabetesinterview.com
Diabetes Self Management	www.diabetes-self-mgmt.com
Endocrine Today	www.endocrinetoday.com
FDA	www.fda.gov/diabetes

Websites

Healthier US Initiative	www.healthierus.gov
Insulin Pumpers	www.insulin-pumpers.org
International Diabetic Athletes Organization	www.diabetes-exercise.org
Diabetes Exercise & Sports Association	1-800-898-4322
Joslin Diabetes Center	www.joslin.harvard.edu
Juvenile Diabetes Foundation	www.jdrf.org (1-800-JDF-CURE)
Medicare Drug Program	www.medicare.gov
Meters	http://www.mendosa.com/meters.htm
NCEP (National Cholesterol Ed Program)	www.nhibi.nih.gov/guidelines/cholesterol/atp3upd 04.pdf.
Nat'l Diabetes Education Program (of NIH & CDC & Prevention in children for health care professionals, parents, school personnel, media)	www.ndep.nih.gov (Small Steps, Big Rewards Program tool kit materials) 1-800-438-5583
National Institute of Diabetes & Digestive and Kidney Disease	www.niddk.nih.gov (1-800-860-8747)
National Diabetes Information Clearinghouse (part of NIH for diabetes patient ed booklets)	www.niddk.nih.gov/diabetes
Online Diabetes Resources by Rick Mendosa	www.mendosa.com/diabetes.htm
The International Diabetes Foundation	www.idf.org unitefordiabetes.org
Weight Control Information Network	www.niddk.nih.gov/health/nutrit/win.htm

Abbreviations

AACE	American Assoc. of Clinical Endocrinologists
AADE	American Assoc. Diabetes Educators
ACE	American College of Endocrinologists
ACOG	American College Obstetrics/Gynecology
ADA	American Diabetes Assoc.
ADA	American Dietetics Assoc.
AHA	American Heart Assoc.
AC/HS	before meals/bedtime
A_{1c}	Glycosylated Hemoglobin (Hb) A_{1c}
A Cell	Alpha cell of pancreas
B Cell	Beta cell of pancreas
BG	Blood Glucose
BS	Blood Sugar
CDE	Certified Diabetes Educator
CGMS	Continuous Glucose Monitoring System
CHD	Coronary Heart Disease
CHO	Carbohydrate
CPT	Certified (insulin) Pump Trainer
CSII	Continuous Subcutaneous Insulin Infusion (Insulin Pump)
CKD	Chronic Kidney Disease
C-Peptide	Connecting Peptide of insulin
DCCT	Diabetes Control & Complications Trial (Type 1)

DKA	Diabetic Keto-Acidosis in Type 1
EDIC	Epidemiology of Diabetes Interventions & Complications
FBS	Fasting Blood Sugar
FPG	Fasting Plasma Glucose
FSH	Follicle stimulating hormone
g	Grams (of Carbohydrate)
GDM	Gestational Diabetes Mellitus (pregnancy)
GLP	Glucagon-Like Peptide (hormone)
HCS	Placental hormone during pregnancy
HDL	High Density Lipo-protein (good cholesterol)
HHS	Hyperosmolar Hyperglycemic State (Non-Ketotic Acidosis)
IDDM	Insulin Dependent Diabetes Mellitus (now Type 1)
IFG	Impaired Fasting Glucose (pre-DM)
IGT	Impaired Glucose Intolerance (pre-DM)
Kg	kilogram (lbs ÷ 2.2)
K cal	Kilo-calorie
LDL	Low Density Lipo-protein (bad cholesterol)
MDI	Multiple Dose Insulin (also basal-bolus)
MNT	Medical Nutrition Therapy
NCBDE	National Certification Board for Diabetes Educators
NIDDM	Non-Insulin Dependent Diabetes Mellitus (now Type 2)
OGT	Oral Glucose Tolerance Test (also GTT)
pc, pp, ppg	Post Prandial (after meal)
PCOS	Polycystic Ovary Syndrome
PVD	Peripheral Vascular Disease
SMBG	Self-Monitoring BG
TDD	Total Daily Dose (of insulin)
Trig	Triglycerides
TZD	Thiazolidindione
UKPDS	United Kingdom Prospective Diabetes Study (Type 2)
U/kg/24 hr	Units/kilogram/24 hours

Oral Medication/Insulins

bid	twice daily
qid	4 times daily
q 2 h	every 2 hours
tid	3 times daily

Apidra (glulisine)

H (Humalog)-LisPro

L (Lantus)-glargine

L (Lente-off the market)

L (Levemir)-detemir

N (NovoLog)-aspart

N (NPH)

R (Regular)

U (Ultra Lente-off the market)

U/hr (Units / hour)

Combination insulins:

Humalog Mix 75/25 (75% N/25% Humalog) Eli Lilly

Novolog Mix 70/30 (70% N/30% Novolog) Novo-Nordisk

Novolin 70/30 (70% NPH/30% Regular) Novo-Nordisk

Humulin 70/30 (70% NPH/30% Regular) Eli Lilly

Humalog 50/05 (50% NPH/50% Humalog) Eli Lilly

Humulin 50/50 (50% NPH/50% Regular) Eli Lilly